DESIGNED TO HEAL

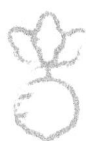 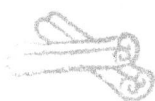 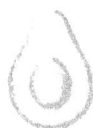

DESIGNED TO HEAL

God's Plan For Our Food, What Went Wrong,
and How to Get Back to It

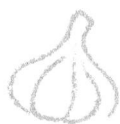 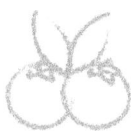 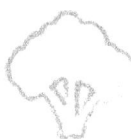 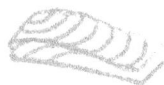

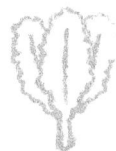 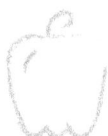 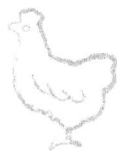 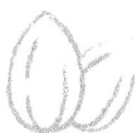

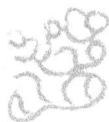 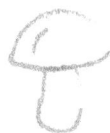  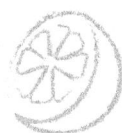

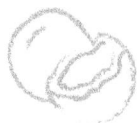 **Alex Morgan**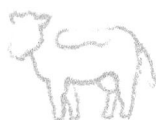

For Haley—your passion for healing will heal many others.

Contents

Foreword

By: David Bruce

Some of my earliest memories of Alex relate to food; more specifically, our high school lunch table. Alex was a classic brown bagger—whole wheat sandwich, fruit, and maybe some Veggie Straws. I was also a classic brown bagger, but I finished my packed lunch by second block and then bought a second one at the cafeteria when actual lunch time rolled around. Our lunch table was the circular kind with eight plastic blue-gray seats and shiny metal support beams that frequently bruised knees trying to shimmy in or out of the seat. While our physical lunch table was everything ordinary, the people and traditions were worthy of a Netflix Original.

We shared a Verse of the Day (VOTD—pronounced "voted"), written on an index card and placed inside Alex's brown bag by his mom every day. After Alex read the VOTD, he would pose the question of the day (QOTD—you guessed it "quoted"), a well-crafted question to which all of us would discuss and debate our answers.

Tuesdays were "Tie Tuesdays," where we all dressed up in tucked-in dress shirts, ties or bow ties, and the occasional sweater vest.

Fridays were "Cookie Fridays," where one person was responsible for bringing homemade cookies. If you're questioning the baking skills of eight 14-year-old guys, we would have surprised you. We rotated the responsibility every week, and it felt more of an honor than a burden to bake cookies the night before. They were frequently delicious. Friday's QOTD took on a special edition, rebranded as "Fist Fight Friday." You might be wondering how eight guys can go from baking cookies to brawling in the same day. No fist fights actually occurred, but rather the QOTD was swapped for something like, "Who would win in a fist fight: Batman or Superman? Tom Brady or Derek Jeter? Dwayne 'The Rock' Johnson or Iron Man?"

Finally, lunch would conclude every day with "The Trash Game." Anyone at the table at any moment during the lunch period would quickly place any item (not just food) above their head, and it was a race for everyone else to put an identical item above their head. The last person to do so would be tasked with taking everyone's trash and red lunch trays to the trash bins. If we didn't have an identical item, we would run throughout the lunchroom to another table and find someone who had the item, take it, and put it above our head. Each table mate was only allowed to initiate the trash game once per week, so if I placed an umbrella above my head on Monday, I'd have to wait until sometime next week to initiate it by placing a plastic spoon above my head. Our lunch table was well-known in the school, probably because the other 1,600 students just wanted our cookies.

My point in sharing all this, aside from how ridiculous it was, is to illustrate that Alex and I have a long-standing relationship around food. And there are countless other food stories from those four years of high school I could share, such as racing to finish a one-pound cheeseburger at Cheeburger Cheeburger (Alex won with a sub-four-minute time) or competing in a doughnut eating competition against a yellow lab (the dog won that one). Food has always had a memorable and important part to play in our friendship, but the most significant food story began when I went all in on a radically different view of food, guided largely by Alex's wife, Haley, in May of 2021.

What prompted my all-in commitment to a lifestyle that dramatically shifted the way I interacted with and thought about food? Well, after almost a year of experiencing bizarre symptoms including bloating, diarrhea, mouth sores, headaches, fatigue, cramps, and losing twenty-five pounds, along with dozens of meetings with doctors, X-rays, ultrasounds, CT scans, MRIs, two upper endoscopies, and a colonoscopy, it was revealed that I had Crohn's Disease. It was a 5:00 p.m. follow-up appointment for the colonoscopy when my doctor said those words, and the next thing I remember her saying was "infusions." Basically, I was told I needed an IV of potent medicine infused directly to my bloodstream every few weeks for the rest of my life. To go from a healthy and athletic 25-year-old who only visited doctors to get a physical for school sports to having a "disease" was a whirlwind. At first, I got behind "attacking this and getting it under control," which was the sentiment by my doctor who strongly encouraged infusions as the treatment plan. Whatever it took to get back to "normal" and not feel awful every single day, I was on board.

Fast forward a few months, I got married and we moved to a new state which delayed starting infusions. Three days before my first infusion appointment, I called and canceled. I had been praying to hear from God about whether I should proceed with infusions, and I never felt peace about it. During this same window of time, Alex and Haley had shared a little bit about food making a difference in their lives. My dad had also suggested I watch a documentary called *Heal*, which details peoples' accounts of chronic diseases being treated by diet. As my wife and I sat in the parking lot one Sunday afternoon about to go grocery shopping for the week, I decided to pivot from all in on infusions to all in on food.

I jumped into the change with hardly any knowledge. All I knew at that point from Alex and Haley was an acronym "SCD" and a photo of a piece of paper from Haley that had typed "Stage 1" and a very brief list of food I could eat. I learned that the Specific Carb Diet (SCD) was all about removing foods that were hard to digest so that your body could detox and heal on real, whole foods. At the start, this was the list of foods to eat: boiled chicken, eggs, green beans, carrots (well-cooked), and sea salt. There were a few other things such as fish, tea, zucchini, and special homemade yogurt, but I'm not a fan of any of those, so I didn't bother. Breakfast, lunch, dinner, and snacks throughout the day consisted of those five things. I was housing 8-9 eggs a day (3-4 for breakfast, 2 for a midday snack, 1 with dinner, and 2 for dessert), along with two Costco-sized packets of organic chicken per day. The result? All my symptoms went away after seven days of this 5-item take on SCD. No exaggeration, I went from seriously sick to symptom free in one week.

That drastic result encouraged me even more to stick with it, and the improvement continued. A few months in, my lab work matched the positive signs I was feeling. My wife and I texted almost daily with Alex and Haley, learning from their experience as I navigated this food journey through each stage of SCD (where, thankfully, you get to add more foods throughout the process). After ten months on the diet, I had a colonoscopy scheduled to really see how things were looking inside. As my gastroenterologist put it, "Just because you're feeling well doesn't mean much has necessarily changed with your Crohn's." Contrary to his belief, the results of the colonoscopy were great—no signs of active Crohn's involvement. With this, my doctor said infusions were not necessary.

Hopefully, you don't need to go as drastic as I did, and I can't promise such quick results, but Alex and Haley's guidance through this food journey has had a life-changing impact on me, literally. I learned that the medical world wasn't the only path to healing; on the contrary, it was the food I was eating that brought true healing. You don't need a medical diagnosis to give this book a chance to impact your life. The insight and guidance Alex and Haley give have the power to improve your life. Let their words impact your life as they did mine.

–David Bruce

DESIGNED TO HEAL

Our Story of Healing

In the summer of 2015, I found myself in a budding romance with my future wife, Haley. It was a full-blown butterflies-inducing season of summer love. We were in college together at Virginia Tech in Blacksburg, Virginia, and we were also both leaders of a campus ministry called Young Life. Those college years were equal parts ridiculous fun, overwhelming stress, and personal growth for us both individually and together.

Between being full-time students, basically full-time Young Life leaders, and trying to navigate a relationship, we were pretty busy. Food wasn't something that much crossed our minds aside from taste, cost, and convenience. I'm talking unlimited parent-sponsored campus food, hot pockets, Cook Out trays, and boxed mac and cheese. I don't think our dietary habits were particularly *unusual* but that doesn't mean they were particularly *healthy* either. Food was food, and like most of us, we thought of it as primarily either for our sustenance or our enjoyment.

Come spring 2017, we were about to graduate. Of course, that brought with it the addition of some wonderful-yet-weighty conversation topics like marriage, careers, and where to move after college. Stress and excitement levels ran high. The weekend before graduation, Haley started to feel really sick and fatigued accompanied by some very irregular bowel movements. She'd had a history of anxiety attacks and irritable bowel syndrome, so doctor visits weren't out of the ordinary for her. This time she went to a gastroenterologist (basically a gut/digestive system doctor) and got a colonoscopy (yep, the thing that 50-year-old men usually get). The news came; she was diagnosed with ulcerative colitis, or UC.

Basically, the doc said, her colon (which is part of the large intestine) had a number of ulcers on it as a result of continuous inflammation in her gut. We were told this was a chronic issue—something she would have to live with for the rest of her life. The docs said that they didn't know what caused UC. It was probably a mix of genetics and high stress they told her. So just bad luck and living a normal American life. Not very comforting. Being an ignorant college boyfriend, I didn't have much more comfort to offer. It's hard to know what to say when you hear, "This will be the rest of your life and there's nothing you can do about it."

The doctors prescribed Haley some steroids and put her on a daily pill that was supposed to calm the inflammation and make everything better in a jiffy. It seemed to be going fine enough for a bit. We got engaged later that year, planned the wedding, and moved to the D.C. metro area to start our careers. Honestly, at that point, I didn't think about her disease all that much. We got married and headed off to the honeymoon in Mexico. What I didn't know is that our lives were about to change in more ways than one.

What would end up becoming the biggest flare-up of Haley's UC had been slowly building for a couple of months at that point, but the lead up to the wedding hadn't given Haley any time to address what she felt in her body. A couple months after the wedding, in August of 2018, we hit a point of no return. Things continued to worsen, and the doctors switched Haley from her daily pill to an every-other-week injection. The stronger medicine (plus reintroducing steroids) should knock this disease out immediately, we were promised. Again. But she just kept getting worse. Soon enough, doctors had doubled her dosage to weekly injections. Still no improvement. It seemed the only path the conventional wisdom could offer was more of the same.

I had fallen in love with a lively, caring, selfless woman and two months into marriage she wasn't even able to get out of bed because of the crippling pain and exhaustion caused by her disease. I did what I could to care for her, but I had no idea how to help. We cried. We prayed. We asked God why this was happening. It didn't make any sense. We felt helpless. But never hopeless.

On the contrary, Haley was inspired at this point. She had this gut feeling (no pun intended) that this couldn't be how things were supposed to be. Our bodies weren't made to break down like this, especially not at twenty-three years old. Haley and I are both Christians, so we started to pray through what healing might look like in God's eyes. We asked Him to show us His way through this and to use this pain for His glory.

Haley started meeting with a nutritionist and researching natural alternatives to the drugs that only seemed to increase in dosage and decrease in effectiveness. This led to her beginning the Specific Carb Diet (SCD), an eating plan designed to restore digestive health. At the beginning, she'd only eat about five foods in their most easily digestible state (think boiled chicken and steamed vegetables). Over the next few months and years, one by one she added in more options and paid close attention to how her system reacted to each. The foods she did add were only whole, organic, real foods. Most anything that came in a box or bag didn't qualify. Perhaps the most important part was that the diet strictly forbade any refined sugars, dairy, or grains—not just gluten. Haley was as determined as I'd ever seen her to stick to what felt like a last-ditch effort.

The results were astounding. Within a couple months she was feeling the best that she had in years. She started putting back on weight that had drained out of her during the flare-up. She had more energy and life. Heck, we celebrated when she had her first normal bowel movement for the first time since her diagnosis.

It was working.

In fact, about a year later when she got a checkup colonoscopy, her GI doctor said that if this was the first time he'd seen her results, he would never have diagnosed her with UC. Although it wasn't the point, I had started seeing personal results too. I'd been (mostly) eating the same stuff as Haley and I lost twenty pounds without even trying. I found it fascinating that this change in our eating habits had simultaneously caused Haley to gain weight she needed and me to lose it. This lifestyle wasn't just for those with chronic diseases, but even those, like me, who seemed healthy enough. It's almost like our bodies were made to work on real, organic, from-the-ground foods. Incredibly, within three years, Haley had entirely stopped all pharmaceuticals for her ulcerative colitis.

We couldn't have been more elated! We praised God for a miracle. A change in her diet had done what more and more medicine promised (yet failed) to do: put this disease in remission. Once we moved past the excitement of that moment, we started to ask ourselves why this wasn't the first thing we tried. Why didn't the doctors connect what she was eating to how her body was acting? Why don't more people understand how these things are intertwined?

What started as a diet of necessity had turned into a passion. As we dove deeper into healing habits, we wanted to be all in, and we wanted to share it with others. Since we'd seen the results firsthand, it almost felt like a responsibility to share what we'd found. In a world where digestive issues, prescription drug addiction, and mental illness seem unstoppable, we wanted others to see food not as a last-ditch effort like we did at first, but as a proactive healing powerhouse. And that powerhouse was more than just a physical healing, but a mental, emotional, and spiritual one as well.

We had found that our spiritual health was far more wrapped up in our physical health than we'd ever realized. In fact, we began to understand that while Haley's healing was a *supernatural* one, it didn't need to be an *unusual* one. Why not? Because God had laid out a path to healing in His original design of our bodies and the food He gave us.

I am absolutely not the authoritative source on any of this stuff. But I think that's part of what made this book worth writing. I'm just a normal guy with a normal wife who fought through a lot of pain and disease and came out the other side.

I'm also a Christian with a deep conviction that God has a design that He calls us to live within. That design is for all aspects of our lives, not just the "religious" parts. This book is what came out of the intersection of our physical and spiritual lives. It shook me at first and I hope it has an effect on you, too. While I don't believe you need to be a Christian to take something away from this book, I hope that in reading it you see the spark of God's beautiful design throughout.

Just like I don't believe you need to be a Christian to take something away from this book, I also don't believe you need to be in obvious need of healing for this book to be useful to you. Sure, you will likely see your body respond in more dramatic ways if you are struggling with a chronic disease like Haley's example. But even for those of us who are "healthy," it is so vital to support our bodies to thrive in the way they were designed to (more akin to my experience). In reality, our bodies are constantly doing the work of healing on a microscale, and how we support them—or not—will have a major role to play in whether we will eventually have that more urgent need for healing. This is especially true in today's world where toxins and stressors are everywhere. Proactive healing is still healing!

This book is not a textbook. It's not a theological dissertation. It's not a cookbook. My hope is that it scratches the surface of the science, the theology, and the practicality of a new (and yet very old) way of viewing food. Because there is *so much* more than what I've written in these few pages. Many of these topics rightly deserve and have their own full-length books. This book serves as an introduction to God's design for our healing through food. We'll cover how God's good design shows up in our food, where we went wrong, and how we can get back to it. Open your eyes to the wide world of healing eating (and the broader healing lifestyle) and I promise you won't regret it. Let this be the first step of a journey towards flourishing. God has a good design for our food, our healing, and our bodies, and we should fight to live in it.

Part I
God's Good Design

Part I
Introduction

Throughout this book, and especially in Part I, we're going to consider God's design for our bodies, our food, and the subsequent implications for our lives. If you've been around church much, you've likely heard the term *God's design* thrown around some. You may associate it with marriage, the family, or even sex. You may also have assumptions about what it means to be "in God's design" or what the consequences are for walking outside of it. For these reasons, before we begin, I want to provide a definition and a disclaimer.

First, the definition. When I use the word *design*, I mean it in a fairly literal sense: how and why God originally made something. The Oxford Dictionary defines *design* as simply "to do or plan something with a specific purpose in mind." Because God is eternally and perfectly wise, everything He makes is made to bring Him glory. That means that everything is designed with a purpose. In a sense, we should ask the question, "What is God's design for [fill in the blank]" about everything, with the assumption that God's original intention for something is the absolute best way for it to operate. [Fill in the blank] will flourish in God's design.

But how do we know what God's design is? It's not always immediately obvious. The first place to look is the Bible. Secondarily, for this particular subject, we will also consider some basic biology. I chose to look at the Bible because I believe the Bible is God's Word to humanity. Therefore, if He wanted to communicate something directly about His design, He would do it there. I chose to look at basic biology (i.e. the study of life) because I believe that God is our Creator, so if we understand how our bodies (and our foods—which are also alive) work, we can gain some insight into His design for us.

With all this in mind, here is the disclaimer: my intention is certainly *not* to imply that every action outside of what I describe in this book is inherently sinful. When it comes to other topics where we commonly speak of God's design, we have the advantage of many specific teachings in the Word. For example, there are many passages that help us understand not only God's *design* for marriage but also God's *commands* for marriage. Since the topic of marriage includes these specific commands, there is a cleaner line between what is right and wrong for every Christian. However, other topics don't always have this advantage of clear and obvious commands. What we should eat to flourish is an example of a topic in that gray area (though we will briefly touch on Jewish dietary laws in a bit). For topics without clear commands, though, seeking God's design is about pursuing flourishing by understanding how and why God made something. What was His intention and how can that support me today? It's not about whether or not you're sinning. It's about trusting the Author of Life to know the best ways to live our lives.

Paul is surprisingly specific on this topic in relation to food. In his letter to the Romans, he directed these verses towards an apparent sect of the early church that decided for some unknown spiritual reason not to eat meat:

> "Let not the one who eats despise the one who abstains, and let not the one who abstains pass judgment on the one who eats, for God has welcomed him [...] for the kingdom of God is not a matter of eating and drinking but of righteousness and peace and joy in the Holy Spirit."
>
> ROMANS 14:3, 17

Paul is quite clear that telling someone they are sinning for eating something you disapprove of is *itself* sinful. That is not my intention. The Kingdom of God is so much bigger than food. I am not trying to send you on a guilt trip or pass judgment. I am most certainly not connecting what you eat to salvation. Salvation comes by faith in the finished work of Christ on the cross alone. Rather, my intent is to support your flourishing by investigating how God has designed our bodies to thrive. I want this book to help you experience what Paul called "righteousness and peace and joy in the Holy Spirit" by thinking about God's design in an arena of your life that you perhaps haven't considered in the past. So please, as you read, consider God's design as something that will help you flourish and thrive rather than a judgment that you are sinning for not following a set of rules.

To hopefully drive this point home (because I believe it is so important for a productive conversation), consider the analogy of money. Christians are called to be stewards of our money, knowing that it is God's in the end. Legalism would pass judgment on every transaction a person makes—putting each in a box of right or wrong. Life isn't that simple, and God cares about what's happening in our hearts. It is more helpful to look at the overarching patterns of our lives to see how we are stewarding our finances and growing a generous heart. Life is about taking steps on a path towards flourishing. Those steps may include identifying and fighting sinful *motives* of our hearts, but that is different than an overly legalistic categorization of every purchase. Isn't that how God intends our spiritual lives to work? We are continually growing and being shaped to be more like Christ by taking steps on a journey. It's not about blindly following rules but about walking with Him.

In a similar way, this book isn't about passing judgment every time you take a bite. Instead, I want to help us all steward the resources of our bodies, which are also ultimately God's, towards our flourishing. We do that by looking at how God designed our bodies to function and our food to fuel them. That may also bring us to the uncomfortable position of considering potentially sinful *motives* of our heart. The purpose of this book is not to give you a set of rules to follow. Rather than asking, "Is this sinful?", let's ask, "How am I stewarding what He has given me for His glory?"

I believe that God did have a specific plan in mind when He made our food and our bodies. Now let's take a step into discovering what that may be.

Chapter 1
The Healing Nature

What comes to mind when you consider God and healing? Maybe you think about one of the many times that Jesus healed people of blindness or leprosy. Maybe you think about some highly charismatic church service that claims to spontaneously heal people of their diseases. Or maybe it brings to mind years of unanswered prayer.

Humans have desired to be healed as long as we've existed as a species. Wherever there is pain, suffering, disease, or death, there is an equally intense desire for healing. We all long for deliverance from the physical, emotional, and mental pains that we experience. This all makes healing one of the most obvious and popular requests asked of God, whether you're religious or otherwise. If you've ever been in an environment where prayer requests are made known, you've certainly heard too much information about Sally's great aunt in the hospital or little Jimmy's broken arm.

In today's world, healing may be one of the hardest things to genuinely believe God will provide. We certainly struggle to believe that God will spontaneously heal. There's probably a different book to write about that topic, but what really eats away at our faith is when our continuous prayers for healing seem to go unanswered. When we keep pleading for a reprieve from pain, but it doesn't come, we begin to think the only logical explanation is that God either isn't real or doesn't care. Neither of those things are true.

God is a healer. That much is plain to see in His Word. He clearly identifies Himself as Israel's healer in Exodus 15. Healing is the most public part of Jesus' ministry and perhaps the main reason that such large crowds followed Him. In fact, we really have no idea how many people Jesus actually healed. Just look at two verses only a chapter apart from each other in the Gospel of Matthew:

> "That evening they brought to Him many who were oppressed by demons, and He cast out the spirits with a word and *healed all* who were sick."
>
> MATTHEW 8:16

> "And Jesus went throughout all the cities and villages, teaching in their synagogues and proclaiming the gospel of the kingdom and *healing every disease and every affliction.*"
>
> MATTHEW 9:35

Apparently, at least for some amount of time, healing every single sick person He could find was a major part of Jesus' ministry. The authors of the New Testament don't even try to estimate how many people Jesus healed. John 21:25 incredibly states that "the world itself could not contain the books that would be written" if the author tried to write down every healing Jesus performed. If you believe in this God, then you believe He's the same yesterday, today, and tomorrow. He is still an abundant healer.

And that's just looking at God's power to physically heal us. But, boy, does He do far more than that! He offers us a holistic healing centered on the cross of Jesus Christ. We weren't just spiritually *sick*; we were flat out spiritually *dead* in our sins. We were past the point of healing in our own strength. That's why our Good Physician didn't just prescribe us a treatment, but instead He Himself became our healing at the cross. If we humble ourselves to admit that we've sinned and confess Jesus as Lord, we become a new creation spiritually and are promised a new body eternally.

God's healing is holistic, and it is final, but it's not always immediate. We don't experience the full effects of His healing this side of Heaven. We all know that to be true—Christian or not—just by observing reality around us. It could be the daily pain of an autoimmune disease, where your body is quite literally battling itself. Maybe you're fighting off the depression that comes with a chronic diagnosis. Or it could be that you're watching a loved one go through some suffering, and you feel helpless to support them. If you are a believer, you absolutely should rest in the hope of a new creation where one day we will have resurrected bodies that will be free from the diseases of this earth. God will bring us into the fullness of physical healing in that age. That much is certain.

But I also believe that God desires for us to experience some measure of that ultimate healing sooner rather than later as it illustrates the way He has already and will continue to heal us. Plus, He just loves us. We are all His creations, and He even calls believers

His own children. As any good father would, God wants to see us thrive. However, it must be on His terms, not ours.

Although many of us believe that God *can* heal, we tend to think about His power to heal only when the need for it is urgent. God's design is better than that. God's healing nature is so ingrained in His being that when He created us in His image, that healing nature was put in us, too. I mean that literally. Our image-bearing bodies are graciously designed to heal themselves. This is such a simple, yet profound idea to wrap our minds around, especially in the Western world.

Our culture is absolutely terrified of sickness, injury, and disease. In a recent survey, 41.7% of Americans said they were afraid or very afraid of becoming seriously ill and 60.2% felt that way about a loved one getting sick. This survey included options like gun violence, economic collapse, and World War III, but sickness reigned as the second highest fear for Americans.[1] With that fear comes an unhealthy over-reliance on Western medicine. This includes pharmaceutical drugs, surgeries, and other similar interventions. Don't get me wrong, there is certainly a time and place for those things. By the grace of God, someone can survive a traumatic car crash by being medevacked to emergency surgery. However, as with all of God's gifts, when we worship the gift over the giver, we lose ourselves. That is exactly what has happened as our collective fear of sickness and over-reliance on Western medicine has formed a cocktail of dangerous behaviors that has become the norm. In all this, we forget that Western medicine would be of no help had our God not designed the body to heal itself in the first place.

Let's do a quick thought experiment. What if your body *wasn't* able to heal itself? What if it was like a new car that started on day one at the peak of existence and depreciated as soon as it left the lot? What if you still wore all the nicks, bruises, diseases, and injuries you've ever sustained? No matter how healthy you were, you wouldn't be able to last all that long. You'd bleed out from a paper cut, eventually! Let alone a bout with pneumonia or a broken bone. If that's how things worked, we'd effectively be doomed.

Our bodies' innate healing ability is the miracle that we experience every day and usually never give a moment to consider. I know that when my car starts making weird noises, I hope that the next time I turn on the engine, the noises go away, but they never do. That's because man's creations don't have the capacity for healing. But God has engineered His creations with healing in their nature. We are more than the sum of our past sufferings because God's design for our bodies (physically, spiritually, emotionally, and mentally) includes healing. Western medicine can aid this process when absolutely necessary, but it shouldn't be relied on as the source of healing.

One incredible example of the healing nature in us is our immune system. God designed our immune system to be split into two sections: the innate immune system and the acquired immune system. The innate system is there from the day you're born, and it knows how to fight off some of the most killer attacking cells. But the even more amazing part is the acquired immune system—your lifelong immunity catalog. As your body learns to fight off specific diseases, it remembers and effectively eliminates that disease from returning. Instead of diseases weakening and killing us, our immune system is actually designed to strengthen us through them. We don't just return to how we were before getting sick, but we're actually better off for having made it through the attack of that virus or disease. What's more, this is possible because our immune system is just that: a system. It isn't just one organ or type of cell. It is a collection of bone marrow, skin, spleen, blood, lymph nodes, and more that work together to protect and heal us.[2] There is a master plan behind all of this, and it is a direct line to healing.

But none of that removes the very real tension between wanting to believe God will heal and what feels like unanswered prayers. Why is it so hard for us to believe that God will heal us? Because we've asked God before, and He hasn't answered. It's starting to seem like He may never answer.

But what if He has?

What if His answer is far better than we could've hoped?

What if He doesn't give us our quick fix because He's already given us a beautiful healing design to walk in?

What if He's trying to show us that He's already given us everything we need to flourish?

What if He answered and we didn't listen?

These are the questions we should be asking. Certainly, there are other reasons God might not answer a prayer the way we wanted, but one of those reasons we must consider is that He wants to reveal to us the better answer that's always been there. We experience more of God's blessing when we walk in His design in any areas of our lives, so why shouldn't that be true of our physical bodies? Of course, living in God's design is not the easiest path. It's not the most convenient path. It's not the cheapest path. But it is the hopeful path. It is the life-giving path. It is the healing path. And that's exactly how He intended it.

Jesus tells his followers, "Small is the gate and narrow the road that leads to life" (Matt. 7:14). The gate may be narrow, but the destination is worth it. While there are larger implications for that passage, it also directly applies to God's design for healing in our bodies. Living within the parameters of God's design in any area of our lives takes real effort. We don't accidentally become emotionally healthy beings. We don't coincidentally become spiritually healthy beings. Why should we act like that is how health works physically?

I don't believe that God set up humankind to lack what it needed to be healthy and thriving until we invented the antibiotic in 1928 or chemotherapy in 1940. God didn't leave us hanging for millennia until we achieved the scientific aptitude to heal ourselves. There's nothing wrong with new discoveries and advancements in medicine. They can be incredible, helpful, and needed in a lot of circumstances. What I am arguing is that there is a Creator who designed us. It follows that, from the beginning, this Creator also provided the resources we needed to thrive. Second Peter 1:3 explicitly states, "His divine power has granted to us all things that pertain to life and godliness." I would say that physical healing fits in the category of "all things that pertain to life." God gave us what we needed, and in the case of healing, He gave us something really specific: food.

Chapter 2
Food Is God's Medicine

If it's true that God designed our bodies to heal themselves and it's true that God provided everything we needed to thrive as humankind from the beginning, then food is God's homegrown medicine. Food is so foundational to the human experience that God designed us to want it nearly constantly. He even designed us to find pleasure in it. Somewhat surprisingly, that is not the norm across the rest of the animal kingdom. The retail and food services industries combine for 6.2 *trillion dollars* in revenue in the US annually and there are 38,000 grocery stores across the country.[1] Food is a mainstay in our social gatherings, our weddings, and our funerals. It could be used to illustrate the human experience.

Have you ever thought about why God set it up that way? What was the point of us needing to chew and swallow hundreds of times a day in order to stay alive? God could've set up the universe in whatever way He wanted to, and that's how He decided to do it.

Part of the answer is that our need for food humbles us. It is a nearly constant reminder that we need something outside of ourselves to survive another day. In fact, the Bread of Life is one of the names God uses for Himself to help us understand our daily need for Him. That need also distinguishes us from God. He doesn't need anything outside of Himself to continue being God, but we can't last more than a month or so without food (and even less without water).

Another reason is that food serves as a way to express some of the deepest emotions. It's not a coincidence that the second coming of Christ comes with a feast or that the return of the prodigal son came with the father serving the fattened calf. Celebration and a good meal go hand in hand. On the flip side, the Bible often pairs fasting with times of sorrow or lament. Refraining from eating was one of the primary ways to show a depth of emotion that words simply could not express.

Those are just a couple of the many spiritually significant reasons that God chose to set up the humans-need-food system the way He did. But there are physical reasons, too. He didn't pick the stuff we're supposed to eat randomly. We don't eat rocks or drink ocean water. Not every food is full of the same nutrients. God picked specific parts of His creation for specific reasons to be the food that sustains our physical bodies.

The more time you spend considering the true God of the Bible, the bigger and higher your view of Him will grow. A high view of God believes that He is sovereign, that He has a good design, and that He doesn't leave us to our own devices to survive in this world. A high view of God doesn't leave room for a high view of man along with it. (See John 3:30, "He must increase, but I must decrease.") This means we should view the creations of God as higher than the creations of man. Mountains are more impressive than bridges. The brain is more brilliant than AI. Space is more immersive than virtual reality. Naturally, this high view of God should lead us to a high view of the food that He made for us. We know that God directly designed our bodies *and* our food. Those are two important pieces to His larger, good design. When humans create something, at best it builds off of God's original design and at worst it perverts it in a way that harms more than helps.

God's original design for food is something that is both ancient wisdom and the ongoing discovery of today's scientists. One of the simple joys in life is seeing a CNN headline that says something akin to "New Study Shows Apples Are Good for You." Had you asked any of our ancestors, they could've told you that! Still, seeing science unearth the details of just how God worked it all together for our good is exhilarating. For example, God designed food with different color schemes for a reason. Foods with similar colors typically have similar nutrients, and we need the full range of those nutrients to nourish our entire system. Orange foods support the spleen and digestive system. Red foods support heart and brain health. Dark blue foods support your kidneys and bladder.[2] From the beginning, these colors have been native all over the world. Avocado, pineapple, and raspberries are native to the Americas. Cherry, elderberry, and carrots are native to Europe. Watermelon, clementine, and dates are native to Africa. Mango, guava, and pitaya are native to Asia. There are so many beautiful colors across our beautiful world.

Not only did God pick His colors with a purpose, but He picked His shapes, too. Oftentimes in nature, the shape of the food directly supports the organ that it resembles. Ginger supports the stomach, celery supports the bones, tomato supports the heart, walnuts support the brain.[3] God had a plan when He designed this world. It is an ordered plan that leads us towards what is nourishing.

God filled our world with so many types of nutrient-rich options for our flourishing: fruits, vegetables, livestock, fish, poultry, eggs, mushrooms, herbs, nuts, seeds, algae, and more. In their natural state, each of these is filled to the brim with a unique mix of micronutrients (vitamins and minerals) that our bodies depend on to thrive. Even in tiny amounts, these micronutrients activate our immune system, signal cell growth, generate hormones, form red blood cells, support wound healing, develop DNA, metabolize food, and produce energy (just to name a few).[4] They are integrated into essentially every possible function of our bodies. Even though these micronutrients are clearly so essential to human flourishing, our bodies can't produce many of them on their own. Do you know where God designed us to get them? Our food.

In our modern world, we've lost a lot of this big vision of God's design for what food is meant to look like. Specifically, we've misdefined food and misunderstood its purpose. By "misdefined" I mean that we call just about anything food. If you can ingest it, you can call it food. This often includes artificial chemicals, additives, and preservatives that don't come from nature. They weren't specifically designed by God to make our body work optimally. Instead, they are the creation of man for our own purposes. Just take a look at maltodextrin and monosodium glutamate, two of the "ingredients" in Cheetos. Seen those growing on a tree recently?

You might be asking yourself, "Well, how am I supposed to know what God's vision for food looks like?" I'm glad you asked. In fact, God actually used the 29th verse in the entire Bible to define, in His words, what food looks like. And might I add, this is even before sin (and subsequently death) had entered the world. This is unequivocally what God intended for us:

> "And God said, 'Behold, I have given you every plant yielding seed that is on the face of all the earth, and every tree with seed in its fruit. You shall have them for food.'"
>
> GENESIS 1:29

And before you say that this means we're all supposed to be vegetarians, God updated this a few years later in His covenant ceremony with Noah:

> "Every moving thing that lives shall be food for you. And as I gave you the green plants, I give you everything."
>
> GENESIS 9:3

That "everything" at the end of that verse is referring to all His living creation, adding animals to the plants God gave to Adam. The point being (and I think this is something we all inherently know to be true) that God created plants and animals, in part, to be the food that fuels us. He gave them to us in their natural, whole, organic forms.

It isn't inconsequential that Genesis 1:29 comes directly after God gave Adam and Eve the great human mandate to "be fruitful and multiply and fill the earth and subdue it" (Genesis 1:28). It seems that, on some level, God wanted to connect the idea of living out our intended purposes to what we eat. And when we live out our intended purposes, we thrive. Food was always meant to be a bedrock of our flourishing (and therefore our healing). Our bodies work the way they are designed to work when we eat what we are designed to eat. Then, we can live out our God-given purposes to a much fuller extent.

I think it is appropriate here for a bit of an aside addressing Jewish dietary laws, since these are the Bible's most specific commands on the topic of eating. These laws are found primarily in Leviticus 11 and repeated in Deuteronomy 14. Let's consider the culmination of these cleanliness laws:

> "You shall not eat anything that has died naturally. You may give it to the sojourner who is within your towns, that he may eat it, or you may sell it to a foreigner. For you are a people holy to the LORD your God."
>
> DEUTERONOMY 14:21a

Firstly, these laws never claim that the reason they are set forth is for the physical health of the Jewish people, rather that they would be "a people holy to the LORD your God." Secondly, God states that a certain type of unclean animal can be given to a sojourner or foreigner to eat. So, if these laws were primarily about health, it would seem very strange that God would suggest giving something dangerous or unhealthy to those outside the nation of Israel. The best way to understand these laws is that they were always meant specifically for the Jewish people, primarily for displaying them as a people set apart for God. Their purpose was to reflect God's holiness and His people's obedience.

Most importantly, Jesus clearly indicated that all foods were now clean (see Mark 7:19 and Acts 10:15). This seems to confirm the idea that those laws were not primarily about physical flourishing, but they provided a glimpse of the hope of holiness through the One who could actually uphold the law—Jesus Himself. He had fulfilled the true purpose of the law.

With all of that said, it is still interesting to consider the foods that God called clean and unclean for the Jewish people. For instance, it's interesting to consider what God did *not* call unclean. While specific animals were unclean, meat in general was not. Dairy was not unclean. Fish were not unclean. Fruits and vegetables were not unclean. God did not hold back wonderful healing foods from His chosen people!

If you read Leviticus 11, you'll likely notice that the vast majority of unclean animals (for example vultures, eagles, or rats) are creatures that we don't typically eat, anyway. That's because many of them are predators and therefore would eat other animals. This increases the chances of these animals having parasites and diseases. On the flip side, "chew[ing] the cud" (Lev. 11:3) was one of the primary requirements to be a clean animal. These are herbivore, grass-eating animals like cows and lamb, otherwise called ruminants. Ruminants are able to extract incredible amounts of nutrients from a plant as simple as grass due to their multi-layered digestive systems. It seems that, on some level, what our food eats matters to God.

So, the Jewish dietary laws don't directly apply to us today and they were primarily to show the holiness of God's chosen people. Yet, through them we can still catch a glimpse into God's healing design for human flourishing.

Now that we've discussed how we often misdefine our food, let's tackle the other mistake that our culture often makes with food: misunderstanding its purpose. In a majority of today's Western world, there isn't much lack of food. Most of us don't have to worry about where the next meal is coming from in the way most of our ancestors did. While that is certainly a blessing, it also causes us to shift the focus of food's purpose. Typically, we eat to fill or to enjoy rather than to flourish or to heal. Filling and enjoying are not inherently wrong, but they are not the height of what God's perfectly designed foods can offer. The truth is that every bite we take moves us towards a balanced, functioning body or away from one. What we believe food is *for* directly affects the choices we make. If food is for simple pleasure or it's just a necessary nuisance, we're likely to grab what's cheap, convenient, and tastes good. If food is God's gift to us to fuel every cell of our bodies towards healing and flourishing, now we may stop to consider whether what we're consuming is supporting or hindering that beautiful design.

Not sold that food's purpose is for our flourishing? Ask yourself if you'd want any of these benefits:

- Reduced blood sugar
- Reduced cholesterol
- Protection against kidney, breast, and prostate cancer
- Reduced risk of heart attack
- Support of healthy digestion[5]

Those are just some of the benefits...of broccoli. And with no side effects! If a pill could claim those benefits, it would fly off the shelves of CVS. In fact, broccoli (along with most fruits and vegetables) is full of compounds called polyphenols. These guys are powerhouses of healing. They get our lymphatic system moving, which detoxes our bodies and fights off chronic inflammation. Through various studies polyphenols have been shown to fight diabetes, heart disease, cancer, dementia, and even the effects of aging.[6]

In our culture, we've been trained to believe that these sorts of powerful benefits can come only from pharmaceutical drugs. Again, Western medicine and pharmaceuticals can be helpful, and there are times when they are absolutely necessary. If you're imminently dying, Western medicine may very well save your life. But it also treats very specific problems in very specific ways. It's inherently short-sighted with a singular aim. I think that's why we like it so much, though. It's fast and it's precise. Unfortunately, it has its costs. Every drug has side effects, some small and some huge. It's likely the more serious your condition, the more serious the side effects will be. Sometimes we need a new drug to fix the problems caused by the first drug. Sometimes we become so dependent on the drug that we use it long after our original ailment necessitated. If you have a high view of God, it seems natural to question if this is really His intention for us.

God's design is a holistic one. You don't eat asparagus to get rid of a headache or pineapple to put you to sleep at night. But the beauty of living in God's design long-term is that it protects you from far more than any pharmaceutical could ever claim to do. Just look at that list of broccoli's benefits again; it covers quite the gambit of potential health issues (some of which are even potential drug side effects). God's well-designed food does this without compromising your future flourishing. On the contrary, you may actually receive *benefits* you weren't expecting! The original medicine is still the best medicine provided by the Great Physician, the Creator God.

It's important at this point to mention that food isn't the *only* medicine that God gave us. We'll talk in the next chapter about some of the other things that God has provided to help us physically flourish. However, I wholeheartedly believe that food is God's primary means for healing in our bodies. You could exercise every day of your life and have a heart attack in the middle of a 100-mile bike ride. You could sleep eleven hours every night and be horribly fatigued because of a gut imbalance. If you are ignoring what you put into your body, the other inputs won't have their intended effects on your health.

I'd argue that food is at least 70 percent of physical flourishing. Yes, I made up that statistic, but that doesn't mean the point isn't true. Healing is right there in front of us, but we have to get up and take it. It typically isn't a quick fix, which is why it's much better if you adopt this mindset *before* you feel the need for it. You'll avoid a lot of pain that way. Wouldn't it be marvelous if you didn't need the miraculous healing story because you proactively walked in God's beautiful design for our food?

That said, no matter where you are today, the good news is that God hasn't set you up for failure. In fact, He provided everything you needed to thrive from the very beginning.

Chapter 3
How We Used to Live

So, the big idea of the last chapter, and this book really, is that God gave us everything we needed to thrive and heal from the very beginning. We saw that all the way back in Genesis 1:29, even when God was creating us, He was thinking about what we would eat. Now I want to take a moment to expand that paradigm from focusing on food to looking at our lifestyles holistically. Not only did God give us the food that we need to heal and thrive in our physical bodies, but He also designed our lives to be in balance within our world, our community, and our own soul.

I find it to be a helpful thought experiment to consider how the hundreds of generations before the modern world lived. Yes, our modern world looks very different from the ancient world. That can make it challenging to connect with our past. You could argue that more has changed about human living in the past 200 years than the previous 2,000 combined. However, while the circumstances that we live in look dramatically different than those of our ancestors, in reality, the author of Ecclesiastes got it right, stating:

"What has been is what will be,

and what has been done is what will be done,

and there is nothing new under the sun."

ECCLESIASTES 1:9

Basically, even though our circumstances look different, we really share much more in common with the past than we like to think. We get stuck in the same pitfalls and traps as our ancestors. Our challenges, in many ways, were their challenges. Their victories can be our victories if we take a moment to consider what they learned and how they lived. It's arrogance that says we've moved past the ancient ways and now know the enlightened way to live. Rather, we should look back with humility and learn from the ways of those who came before us.

If you still aren't convinced that there's a real reason to look backwards, consider the statistics in rising disease (stats that I bet you could attest to from experience).

Cardiovascular disease is the number one cause of death in the world and has essentially doubled in annual cases since just 1990.[1]

In that same time period, cases of depression have risen 50 percent.[2]

When immunology began being studied in the early 1900s, the idea that your immune system may attack itself to the point of disease was ludicrous. Despite some evidence, the idea of autoimmune disease was fought until the 1960s when the evidence became overwhelming.[3]

In 1996, an estimated 8.5 million Americans suffered from an auto-immune disease.[4] In 2019, that number was more than 50 million.[5]

The CDC says that 6 in 10 adults in the U.S. have a chronic disease and 4 in 10 have two or more.[6]

Something isn't working in our so-called enlightened humanity. Disease and death are increasing despite the most sophisticated medical advancements the world has ever seen. It seems logical that there is something wrong with the way we're living. So, what are some of the big differences between our lives and those of our ancestors? I'm glad you asked.

The logical first place to look is food. What did the ancients eat? Well, whatever they could grow, kill, or gather. The idea here being that they ate straight from the ground or straight from the source. And guess what? Their produce was all local, organic, and never genetically modified. Their meat was always grass-fed and pasture-raised. Those aren't fads meant to steal a couple extra bucks from your wallet. They're actually the way that humankind ate for millennia because pesticides, soy-based animal feed, global supply chains, and genetically modified foods simply didn't exist.

Ancient diets couldn't include processed snacks, bleached flours, and canola oil. Instead, they would be filled with in-season green plants, fresh meats, fruits, nuts, and seeds. And their preparation methods were simple, such as eating raw, roasting over a fire, boiling in water, or fermenting for longevity.

Another vital difference was that our ancestors didn't face the almost overwhelming levels of chemical contamination that we quite simply can't avoid today. Their water, dirt, air, produce, meats, and homes were what we'd now call non-toxic. This would've allowed healthy bacteria and probiotics to support super-charged immune systems.

Not to mention, they had to work for their food. And by work, I don't mean driving to Kroger. They were active people. Constantly moving. Always on their feet because that is simply what life demanded. If they wanted to go to the next town over, they spent half the day walking there. If they wanted food, they got out there and farmed or hunted it. Their activity and movement weren't for vanity's sake; it was for survival's sake. When they were moving, they were moving *outside*. They would get hours of sunlight a day, which is connected with both physical and mental healing. This one hit hard personally as someone who has done the work-from-home, sit-for-8-hours-straight life. Our bodies were designed to move. A lot. We don't always feel that way when we live mostly sedentary lifestyles with largely concentrated spurts of movement.

Importantly, this constant movement was almost always with *other people*. Ancient communities were uniquely social people out of a level of necessity that we couldn't begin to understand. They had a community bond that was life or death. That bond and their intimately shared experiences meant sharing laughter, fear, anger, sadness, and joy with other human beings. They wouldn't have felt isolated. They had their families or tribes. They didn't need to scroll through their social media apps to keep track of what was happening in others' lives because they lived life *with* their community. Isn't it telling that though our world is more "connected" than ever, the rates of loneliness and depression are skyrocketing?[7] Our ancestors were inherently focused on the tight-knit group of family and friends directly around them because that was their only option. But that didn't hold them back; in fact, it may have been one of their greatest strengths.

So, the ancients would eat fresh, local, whole foods and be moving all day. But what if they couldn't catch anything? Or what if their crops were eaten by a wild animal? Something else the ancients understood far better than our modern society was the value of fasting. They often wouldn't eat three square meals a day, simply because they couldn't. But they would also *voluntarily* fast out of spiritual need far more often than the typical Westerner today.

Fasting has tremendous spiritual value; it humbles us and symbolizes our deep dependence on God's provision in our lives. But God also gave it to us as a physical gift. Fasting is a cellular pause where our bodies can truly rest and digest. When our body doesn't need to expend energy metabolizing food, it will use that energy towards creating new, healthy cells. Unhealthy, dangerous cells are simultaneously starved without their normal serving of glucose. Together, this brings a type of healing that we otherwise couldn't experience. Praying for healing must have been one of the main reasons our ancestors would fast. The crazy thing is that God would use the actual act of fasting to begin that healing in them. Just even more evidence that God designed this whole thing called life!

Besides fasting when they were awake, the ancients did a lot more of another type of fast: sleep. They couldn't do much after dark, so their bodies were in tune with the cycle of the sun. They would sleep at dark and rise at dawn following the changing of the seasons for full, restful, healing sleep. The less than seven hours that a third of adult Americans get per night doesn't count as a full night's rest.[8] Our ancestors would get upwards of eleven hours of sleep. Heck, even as recently as 1910, the average American slept nine hours per night.[9] This is one area that we particularly struggle with as a modern culture because the sun going down doesn't really change much for us. We can still work and play without nature's light. We're tempted to never stop because we don't have the built-in limitation. However, sleep is so important for the same reason as fasting: once our body truly rests, healing can begin.

Even in our waking life, rest is such a necessity that it's no wonder God separated an entire day for it. He hard-wired our bodies to function correctly only if we've fought to rest. The ancients didn't have to try nearly as hard as we do to rest because their lives were naturally slower than ours. They'd walk from place to place, not drive. They didn't wear watches or keep schedules (at least not the way we over-stuff ours). They certainly weren't addicted to Instagram. I can only imagine the attention spans they must've had. When people asked them how they were doing, the default answer wouldn't have been "busy." Their lives were simpler and that's not a bad thing. They followed the rhythms of nature, their bodies, and their communities. Their lives were much more singularly focused instead of the multitasking rubber-band balls of lives we often live.

I think you probably get the point by now. The ancients lived slow-paced, communal, naturally active, whole-food-filled lives that looked a lot different from ours, but that doesn't mean the principles of their lifestyle are unobtainable. While, granted, they also faced death in ways we don't understand (ravaged by wolves, anyone?), they would be equally shocked by the epidemic of disease that has become normal even in our modern medicine-filled world. I'm no historian, and this may be a somewhat romanticized look at the past. However, if you take an honest assessment of the state of health in our time, you can only conclude that we're missing something. I'm suggesting that maybe the answer for the way forward can be found by taking a peek back.

Chapter 4
Balancing Act

What do diabetes, cancer, obesity, arthritis, allergies, and a stroke have in common? Way more than you might think. In answering that question, we'll dive deeper into one of the biggest pitfalls of Western medicine—the idea that each diagnosis is siloed and needs its own very specific cure. We get so laser focused on the diagnosis and treatment of a specific infirmity that we lose the bigger picture. Again, I understand how we got here. The promise of Western medicine is a quick fix to your specific problem. But even Western medicine knows there are deeper links between infirmities than we've been led to believe.

For instance, take a look at Humira, the injection my wife, Haley, was prescribed for her ulcerative colitis. That same medicine can be used to treat UC, Crohn's disease, ankylosing spondylitis, plaque psoriasis, and arthritis. Those diseases affect the colon, the small intestine, the spine, the skin, and the joints, respectively. How can the same medicine work on so many diseases affecting vastly different parts of your body? The answer is the *root cause*.

So, what do all those health issues at the beginning of the chapter have in common? In a word: *inflammation*. Every one of those diseases is linked to inflammation in the body. What a harmless-sounding word. When I first understood that Haley's UC was primarily an issue of an inflamed colon, I couldn't quite grasp the why that was such a problem. So, your colon is a little puffy, what's the big deal? Don't body parts get inflamed when there's an issue and then go back to normal after a day or two? Like a bee sting or a bruise?

Well, yes, that's exactly what's supposed to happen. Inflammation is one of our immune system's key responses to invaders (anything that isn't supposed to be there, such as mold, heavy metals, excess blood, parasites, or a number of other things). When our immune system senses an issue, it will put on its natural armor of inflammation, expel the intruder, and get back to normal business. Easy enough.

But what happens if we are continually introducing invaders into our body? What if our dynamic, life-supporting immune system never gets to rest? That is when we move from *acute* inflammation to *chronic* inflammation. Our immune system becomes a city under siege, where even the strongest walls eventually fall.

At that point, our immune system isn't able to separate the functioning, healthy parts of our body from the intruder, and so it attacks itself. We've now entered into disease. That harmless-sounding word, *inflammation*, can lead to horrifying and deadly conditions such as cancer, stroke, diabetes, and more.

I'm not the only one saying this. In fact, it's essentially medical consensus, even if you've never heard of it. Just read this quote from research done by a Ph.D. fellow at the National Institutes of Health:

> "Although chronic inflammation progresses silently, it is the cause of most chronic diseases and presents a major threat to the health and longevity of individuals."[1]

Read that again.

Inflammation is the *cause* of:

Most. Chronic. Diseases.

Shouldn't we be ringing alarm bells about this thing? Shouldn't everyone know about this? It's not a mystery why our immune systems turned against us. We have real insight into why our bodies have started to attack us instead of heal us.

Chronic inflammation is a civil war in our bodies culminating in chronic disease. Our body is quite literally attacking itself.

That's what autoimmune disorders are—your immune system attacking healthy cells instead of sick ones.

That's what cancer is—your cells destructively refusing to stop making more of themselves.

That's what diabetes is—your cells ignoring the signals sent by insulin to convert glucose into energy.

That's what allergies are—your body deciding that something (typically) harmless is actually harmful.

Chronic inflammation leads to our body working against itself because it has lost the ability to distinguish the good from the bad, helpful from harmful. We've forced our immune system to work so hard for so long that its walls have collapsed. We're defenseless.

So, the next logical question should be clear. If so much hinges on whether or not we are experiencing chronic inflammation, what causes that level of chronic inflammation? At least one of the major causes is imbalance in your gut.

What do I mean by that?

I mean that within our gastrointestinal tracts (primarily upper and lower intestines) there lives a microscopic environment of trillions of bacteria. It's called the gut microbiome and it's so important that some are starting to label it as an organ.[2] This collection of bacteria plays a major role in at least our metabolism, immune function, and communication between our body and our brain.[3] Since the microbiome is a relatively new discovery, we're still constantly learning more about the massive role it plays in our bodily functions.

One thing we do know is that the microbiome is sort of like Star Wars—there's a battle between the light bacteria and the dark bacteria. Harmony happens when there is balance in the biome. What throws it out of balance is the fact that bad bacteria are prone to overgrowth if not controlled. When one strand of bacteria begins to dominate, it reduces the microbiome's diversity, which in turn reduces its effectiveness in supporting digestion and immune function. This leads to inflammation. We want our gut bacteria to exist together in harmony, with no specific strand dominating the others. This only happens if the good bacteria are strong enough to regulate the bad.

Everything that we put into our bodies is either helping move towards balance or away from it. The bad bacteria feed heavily on ultra-processed foods, especially those that contain high amounts of refined sugar.[4] The good bacteria feed off fibers found mostly in vegetables and some fruits and whole grains. Besides food, the microbiome can be thrown out of balance by pharmaceuticals such as antibiotics or steroids, pesticides from non-organic food (or our front yard), and contaminated drinking water. All of this can have serious effects on the delicate balance of our gut and therefore chronic inflammation in our bodies.

Sometimes we can't control the things that are affecting our microbiome. There are external factors that we simply can't change that may have a negative effect on our well-being. But this is all the more reason we need to be actively supporting the good bacteria.

In today's toxic world, if we aren't *in* the fight for balance, then we are losing it. The typical American diet is much more likely to be feeding the bad bacteria than the good. While our ancient ancestors may have been able to be in balance while living within their cultural norms, in this day and age it is next to impossible to accidentally have a balanced gut. It must be an active fight.

When the gut becomes imbalanced, immune cells activate against the bad bacteria, causing inflammation to fight these intruders in our system. This wouldn't be a problem in an isolated event, but when we keep eating the same foods, taking the same medicines, and drinking the same water that caused that initial inflammation, then the immune system continues to attack and inflame, attack and inflame. This inflammation starts to affect us at a cellular level by decreasing our Regulatory T cells. Without those T cells, our immune system gets confused and refuses to turn off when it should.[5] All of this keeps compounding on itself until our chronic inflammation becomes full-on *disease*.

Of course, balance in the microbiome is not the only thing affecting our long-term health, but the microbiome is central to our healing. It has connections to massive players such as hormone production, insulin sensitivity, lymphatic flow, healthy sleep, and stress levels, just to name a few. Your body won't flourish if you are focusing on the symptoms alone, but once you get to the root cause of your infirmity, true healing can actually begin. Inflammation and imbalance in our gut are some of the most common underlying root causes to consider. When you focus on fighting these root causes, each of the interconnected systems of your body can begin to simultaneously support and be supported.

The point isn't simply to understand the microbiome, but to open our eyes to the indescribable interplay and cross-regulation that happens throughout the body. I mean, isn't it stunning to know that there are trillions of bacteria living in the ecosystem of your body, helping you heal and thrive without you even knowing it? God knows every single one of those bacteria by name. He designed us so intricately that scientists are discovering massive things about our bodies all the time. We have an unfathomably creative God. He is as awe-inspiring and intentional as He is loving and good.

Learning more about how our bodies work gives us motivation and focus to treat them right, but it also reinforces the need to trust the Creator. He is the only one who knows every detail and every interconnection. He knit us together in our mother's womb. He seeks our good, so we can trust that He set up His system to work for our healing.

God's good design isn't an accident. In His wisdom, He set it up so that whole, natural, organic foods provide balance to our bodies. Often, the foods we already know to be "bad for us" drive imbalance. The problem is that we often don't feel the full impact of the day-to-day poison we put in our bodies until it is made abundantly obvious in disease.

God designed our bodies to heal and flourish. He also gave us the medicine to do it. Even in the worst of circumstances, you aren't doomed to remain in a state of imbalance forever. The more you arm yourself with knowledge of God's design, the more you'll be able to find hope in His plan. Chronic inflammation leading to chronic disease is not our destiny. On the contrary, we're made for freedom and healing through living in God's good design.

Chapter 5
More Than Physical

Most of what we've covered so far has to do with the physicality of our bodies. That is a logical place to start. It's the most obvious way to see and feel the effects of food and lifestyle changes. We started by looking at how God designed our bodies to be able to heal themselves. Next, we saw how God provided the medicine to heal us in the food that He masterfully designed. We've also seen how God intricately designed the inner workings of our digestive system to work for us and not against us. But, while the impact of God's beautiful design for our bodies and our food is not less than feeling physically better, it is certainly much more.

God is involved in our food. And if God is involved, food and our spiritual lives are far more related than we may realize. If we believe in the God of the Bible, then we believe in a God who was intimately involved in our creation and continues to be intimately involved in our lives. All of the world was made for His glory, including our bodies. He didn't design us to desire three meals per day for no reason. He wanted our need for sustenance to remind us of our need for Him. He wanted our need for physical healing to remind us of our need for spiritual healing. He has a design for our eating habits the same way He has a design for the rest of our lives.

If this is true, then it makes sense to take the next step and believe that He has a way for us to interact with food, which leads to flourishing. And if this path to flourishing exists, then so does a path towards destruction. We believe this about other parts of our lives, don't we?

Take work for example (one of God's other pre-sin designs). I think most Christians would typically believe that God has designed us to work and provide for our families. I think most Christians would also agree that there are destructive ways to go about our relationship with work and that when we do it poorly it can negatively affect our spiritual life. If someone is burning the candle at both ends, working 80-hour weeks, and neglecting their family, this is clearly against God's design for work. We can see this both through God's call for us to rest through Sabbath and through the experiential reality of living with the effects of such an overwhelming work week. It clearly does not lead to flourishing.

But I don't see many people, even many mature believers, applying the same principles to our food. Food becomes a routine and, eventually, an afterthought. We don't take the time to think about what we're putting in our bodies, how it affects us, or how it affects our spiritual health.

This needs to change.

Since God has a flourishing path for our interactions with food, we should desire to pursue it. He is the author of life and, therefore, He knows what abundant life looks like. If we choose to follow our flesh's desires rather than His, we cannot thrive spiritually. Consider the story of the Israelites in Numbers 11. Essentially, the Israelites were wandering in the wilderness, and they began to complain that God wasn't giving them the food they wanted. They had been living off of a miraculously provided food straight from Heaven up until this point, but they wanted more. They even got to the point of longing to be back in their slavery in Egypt because they liked the food better there. As God often does to discipline His children, He allowed them to have their sinful desires. They asked for meat, and they got so much of it that it came "out of their nostrils" and "it became loathsome to them" (Numbers 11:20).

While the subject of this story is clearly food, the backdrop is more truly the Israelites' spiritual lives. Food had become a symbol of their lack of satisfaction in God, their selfishness, and their untamed fleshly desire. They couldn't thrive spiritually in this state. They had adopted a way of interacting with food that led to destruction, seen clearly by what it revealed about their hearts.

So then, what is the flourishing path for interacting with food and positively impacting our spiritual lives? The Bible gives both some specifics and some generalities around food that should be helpful in answering that question. Paul teaches us:

> "So, whether you eat or drink, or whatever you do, do all
> to the glory of God."
>
> 1 CORINTHIANS 10:31

This reminder comes after a discussion on whether Christians should eat food that had been offered to pagan idols. Paul makes it clear that it's not necessarily about the food, but about the heart behind it. Why am I eating this? How does drinking this look to others? Am I bringing glory to God by my choices of what to put in my body? And that's a great place to start. God didn't give us a diet plan. What He did was provide us with nourishing foods to help our bodies thrive. So, question number one is, *Does what I am eating and the way I am eating it bring glory to God?*

Answering that question is by no means easy, but we do have some foundations to build on. We know that God is glorified when we are satisfied in Him. It follows then that when given the choice between God-given gifts and a man-made production, being satisfied in His gifts brings Him glory. We also know that He designed us to flourish. It follows then that He is glorified when we trust that within His design is where we will flourish most. There isn't a checklist to bring God glory in how you eat but trusting Him and eating what causes flourishing is a good start. He designed you to flourish. He wants you to flourish. He is glorified when you flourish!

Step one is to seek to bring God glory in our eating. On to step two, where we consider Paul's words to the Galatian church:

> "For the desires of the flesh are against the Spirit, and the desires of the Spirit are against the flesh."
> GALATIANS 5:17a

While this idea has many applications in both our physical and spiritual lives, it certainly applies to food. Where else do we more acutely feel the desires of the flesh than in our stomachs? Haven't we all so often felt that we physically can't stop ourselves from eating that brownie in front of us? Or that third slice of pizza? The foods that are the worst for us are also the most addicting. In a very real way, many of us are addicted to foods that are killing us. We can't *not* have them. We're like the Israelites craving after meat in the wilderness. And often God's response is similar to us as it was then: He allows us to have it until we can realize that it won't satisfy us. If we are in a place where we *need* something besides God to feel satisfied, we have not offered Him that part of ourselves, and our spiritual lives suffer for it. We have lived out Paul's warning to the Philippians:

> "Their end is destruction, their god is their belly, and they glory in their shame, with minds set on earthly things."
> PHILIPPIANS 3:19

Maybe you've struggled to treat your body as the temple that God dwells in, even if you intellectually think you should. Maybe it's not that you don't have the drive or the time. Maybe there are deep-rooted motivations that become blind spots to sin (potentially the ones we'll talk through in Part II). I'm not saying this is definitely the case for you, but it is worth at least considering for the sake of your soul. Certainly, these blind spots can go both ways. An unhealthy obsession with "healthy" eating (ironic because, at this point, it isn't healthy at all) can be motivated by just as ugly of desires. It's not just what you're doing, but why you're doing it that matters. In either case, the second question to ask is, *In the category of food, am I in bondage to my flesh?*

As we grow in our spiritual lives and understand the depths of love and intimacy that God has shown us through His Son Jesus, those two questions should resound in every aspect of our lives. How am I glorifying God in this? Am I in bondage to my sin and flesh? Or asked a different way, *How can I break the chains of sin in my life and seek to glorify Him in everything I do?* The more our eyes are opened to His love, the more we are compelled to respond in that way.

The beauty of God's plan with food (and really in any way we pursue His design) is that it touches every aspect of our lives. Aside from the physical and the spiritual that we've already discussed, pursuing God's design for food significantly affects our mental and emotional lives as well. Remember the microbiome we talked about in the last chapter? Well, those beautiful, good bacteria are also key in producing serotonin, the neurotransmitter that regulates our moods, sleep, and appetite, among other things. Ninety-five percent of the body's serotonin is made in the gut.[1] On top of that, an amino acid called glycine (which is found mostly in high quality, unprocessed animal fats) stimulates the gut to produce that serotonin.[2] If the bad bacteria are winning the battle and the gut is out of balance (from high refined sugars, ultra-processed foods, etc.), then your body is not adequately making your serotonin.

Put plainly: you won't feel happy.

But if you're living in God's original design for food, your emotions will be in a much healthier balance.

Over the last decade or so this connection has been investigated as the U.S. has plunged into an epidemic of depression, anxiety, and mental health disorders. Drew Ramsey, an assistant clinical professor at Columbia University says, "The risk of depression increases about 80% when you compare teens with the lowest-quality diet, or what we call the Western diet, to those who eat a higher-quality, whole-foods diet."[3] His research has also shown that ADD risk doubles with the Western diet. Some have even dubbed the gut the "second brain" because of the intense connections between our mental health and our microbiome health.

Hopefully, by now the connections are clear (and these are just a couple examples). The point of the whole first part of this book is to get you thinking about food in a new way. Trying to force yourself to diet in order to lose a few pounds hardly ever works for long. However, learning about the ways that food interacts with your body, your brain, and your spiritual life can radically change the way you approach your meals every day. It can change your desires, not just your behaviors.

Food is the fuel that keeps us running either towards or away from flourishing. It touches every aspect of our being.

Your body cares about what you eat.

Your brain cares about what you eat.

Your soul cares about what you eat.

Most importantly, God cares about why you eat it.

We can choose what kind of fuel we put into our bodies. If you put diesel into a gas-powered car, things come crashing to a halt pretty quickly. It's the same with our bodies. If we replace the masterfully-designed, nutrient-dense, organically-real foods that God graciously gave us to eat with the over-processed, chemical-covered, sugar-filled foods of the typical Western diet, things fall apart. On the contrary, if we trust in His perfectly designed foods for our perfectly designed bodies, we flourish.

As we conclude the first part of this book, I recognize that this way of viewing food is very counter-cultural. It's natural to wonder why our Western world bristles against the idea of food as healing. That's exactly what we'll tackle in Part II. It's vital to have a clear view of the forces battling against us if we have any chance of living out this new (and yet very old) understanding of food. That battle can be difficult, but that doesn't mean it's impossible. And living in God's good design is always worth it.

Part II
What Went Wrong?

Part II
Introduction

If God designed our bodies to heal themselves and He gave us food as the primary method for our healing, then what went wrong? Clearly, the state of physical, mental, and emotional health in the Western world is not living out this good design. Surely God meant us for more than the insane rates of chronic disease, obesity, inflammation, imbalance, fatigue, mental illness, and more that plague our culture. These chronic, painful, life-altering diseases have wreaked havoc on our societies. *At best*, you have a second-hand account of chronic disease or other unexpected health deterioration. More likely, you have your own personal account that shows the stark disconnect between the good design of Part I and the reality of this world.

We know what it feels like to live a life where our bodies are working *against* us, not *for* us.

We know what it feels like to be so *used to* the pain that we *don't even realize* our bodies are failing us.

We *know* that something is wrong.

So, what gives? What is the gap between the *design for* and *reality of* our bodies? In a single word, the answer is sin. It's the churchy answer, I know. But it's still absolutely the right answer. The middle third of this book will explore this answer more thoroughly.

Have you ever thought about how the first sin in human history happened while eating?

> "So when the woman saw that the tree was good for food,
> and that it was a delight to the eyes, and that the tree was
> to be desired to make one wise, she took of its fruit and
> ate, and she also gave some to her husband who was with
> her, and he ate."
>
> GENESIS 3:6

Back in the Garden of Eden, where God made every green plant for Adam and Eve's well-being, God made a rule about what not to eat. In fact, God *only* made a rule about what not to eat. From the very beginning, on some level, there was a connection between what we put in our bodies and how we honor God.

The serpent that tempted Adam and Eve in the garden was quite deceptive, or as Genesis coins it, *crafty*:

> "Now the serpent was more crafty than any other beast of
> the field that the LORD God had made."
>
> GENESIS 3:1a

The serpent used Adam and Eve's appetites against them. God gave them their appetites, so the desire for good food was not the problem. The issue came when the serpent convinced them to place that appetite above what God Himself had called them to. The serpent used a deceptive practice to misorder their appetites.

That hasn't changed today. The devil convinces us to place our flesh's appetites in front of God's design for our flourishing. Sin is so tempting because the things that are offered to us are usually good things which the devil convinces us are the most important things. He can't force us to sin, but he can lie to us about what's important. The tempter's primary method is to lure and entice us with our own desire, as James 1:14 tells us.

In other words, we have misordered our appetites.

We become convinced that we'd be lost without "it" (whatever "it" is), when in fact it's quite the opposite. Whether it's food, sex, money, etc., we sin because our desires are not in the appropriate order. The consequence of sin has always been a severed relationship with the Creator. And when the relationship with the Creator is severed, our ability to live in His good design is greatly diminished.

What that means on a personal level is that we each need the blood of Christ to cover us to restore that relationship with our Creator. The implication on a societal level is that our world as a whole has been marred by the dramatic effects of sin. This produces an environment that makes it incredibly challenging to live out God's good design, but not impossible. To take steps to live it out, though, we need to identify our potential blind spots to sin.

What Went Wrong?

That's exactly what we'll explore in the upcoming chapters. We'll consider how sin has corrupted our experience with food via misordered appetites that are played to by deceptive practices. In Adam and Eve's case, there were three seemingly benevolent desires that were ultimately misordered appetites: the forbidden fruit seemed "good for food," "a delight to the eyes," and "desired to make one wise." The serpent used the deceptive practice of twisting God's words to prey on those misordered appetites. Those three desires still haunt the human race. In the realm of eating, they show up as three modern obsessions, which on the surface seem benevolent, but left unchecked can become misordered appetites played to by deceptive practices. Those desires are convenience, taste, and cost.

Since Jesus told us not to pick out the speck in our neighbor's eye and miss the plank in our own, it only seems right to start this part of our journey by looking inward. Have you ever stopped to ask yourself why you eat what you eat? Pause for a second and think about it right now. Why did you eat what you ate for dinner last night or breakfast this morning?

If you're anything like, well, most anyone, then it was some combination of how easily you could get your hands on it, how good it tasted, or how much it cost. If you went to Chick-Fil-A, it may have been all three of those reasons. And on the surface, those reasons seem fine enough. I mean, who has time to cook? Why deprive yourself of some finger-lickin' fried chicken? And seriously, can you beat that deal? Any of those questions sound familiar?

The problem starts to emerge when we contrast Part I (God's Design) with that thought process or when we ask ourselves, "How does God intend for me to interact with food?" Well, if He really designed food to be the fuel for our lives and for the physical, mental, emotional, and even spiritual healing power that we talked about, it would also make sense that He intended us to thoughtfully interact with our food. He wants us to eat foods that nourish our body and allow our body to work at its full potential. But as we do in any other arena of our lives, we far too often usurp the good, God-given design with our misordered appetites played to by deceptive practices.

In Part II, we'll look at those three appetites (convenience, taste, and cost). For each, we'll start by considering how it can become a misordered appetite. Then, we'll consider how deceptive practices can prey on our already misordered desire. As we consider the problem, remember that the only way to break sin's grip is by bringing it to the light. That is exactly what these chapters are meant to do. Opening your eyes to the problem is the first step to overcoming it.

Chapter 6
Chasing Convenience

If you could boil down the rally cry of the twenty-first century to a word, it would have to be *convenience*. It's all about getting what you want, when you want it. For Eve, she saw the forbidden fruit and thought it was "good for food" even though God had told Adam quite the opposite. It was, in fact, the only fruit in the garden that was not "good for food." When our eyes are focusing on the wrong thing, we can take things that were not designed for our good and put our own self-proclaimed *good* label on them. In that vein, when we overemphasize convenience in our diets, we mimic Eve's misordered appetite by saying that something is good *enough* for food. We lower our quality standards to meet our convenience standards. Sometimes, maybe oftentimes, we have to choose between the two. And in today's world, is convenience ever going to lose that battle?

Convenience's favorite buzzword is *efficiency*. Efficiency is all about reducing waste, and in most of our lives that means reducing wasted *time*. All you need to do is look at the popularity of Amazon two-day delivery, ChatGPT, and Roombas to get a glimpse of our desire to gain daily efficiencies. We feel the need for these efficiencies because our Western culture preaches us a message that we should all be working ten-hour days to get that promotion, taking our kids to twelve sports practices a week, working out five days a week, volunteering on the weekends, and watching the latest HBO release. For that to be even remotely possible, we need to "optimize" some part of our schedule to reduce "waste." What that usually ends up translating to is mealtime. Maybe that looks like grabbing fast food on the way home from practice, Uber Eats to the office, or a protein bar after a couple hours at the gym.

There isn't anything wrong with not wanting to waste time; we should steward our time well. In fact, I'm an industrial engineer by trade, where optimizing systems is one of our primary roles. But a few questions then arise: How do we define *wasted* time? What is *valuable* time? When it comes to food, our culture teaches us to assume that convenience is always better. The underlying assumption with that mindset is that time spent eating is wasted time. Eating is a necessary nuisance that should be minimized. But is that true?

For one, our ancestors certainly wouldn't have considered mealtime a waste. It was the primary practical mission of their life to find, prepare, serve, and enjoy meals together. A vast majority of people worked in the agricultural world. When they went to work, it was for the sake of food. Food wasn't a trivial nicety to be minimized; it was on the forefront, not only out of necessity for survival but also for the sake of community. This was intentional. The table has a special place in God's design because it is the centerpiece of the gathering of a family.

God has a family. He gathered them in the Old Testament around seven scheduled feasts every year. Jesus ate with those He sought to know more, and He gathered His disciples for one last supper before He died. Christians are called to remember Christ's cross often through the Lord's Supper. The early church dedicated themselves to the apostles' teachings, prayer, and breaking bread together in fellowship. Ultimately, God will gather His family at a marvelous wedding feast.

Jesus tells a parable about this final banquet in Luke 14. In this parable, three of the invited guests give excuses as to why they can't come. The first says he bought a field and needs to go out and see it. The second says he bought a group of oxen and needs to examine them. Finally, the third had just been married and that was reason enough for him not to join. One of the points of this parable was that, even in Jesus' day, people were too busy to come to the table. They were too distracted to make space for a slow but brilliant meal. Too "optimized" to see what really mattered. Of course, what really matters in this parable is the Kingdom of God, but I don't think it's inconsequential that the Kingdom is visualized as a great meal. In Revelation, Jesus again invites us to a meal:

> "Behold, I stand at the door and knock. If anyone hears
> my voice and opens the door, I will come in to him and
> *eat* with him, and he with me."
>
> REVELATION 3:20

Isn't it somewhat surprising to our Western ears just how often God uses the imagery or even the literal dinner table for His purposes? For something that we've relegated to an afterthought, God brings to the limelight. God certainly has more in store for our meals than streamlined calorie intake. He's designed the table as a place for community, conversation, and life to happen. Devastatingly, one estimate says that only about 30% of American families eat together regularly.[1] That's less than a third of the country's population having daily, set-aside time to engage with their loved ones. Real, meaningful conversations are simply happening less often when meals are focused on convenience rather than purpose.

Besides the negative impacts on our communities, our convenience-focused meals can have a direct impact on our physical health, as well. When we seek convenience in our meals, that usually means two things. First, it likely means that our schedules are so filled to the brim that these convenient meals are necessary. This kind of packed schedule almost always brings with it high levels of stress. Stress is truly one of the worst things we can do to our bodies. According to the American Psychological Association, stress can affect our musculoskeletal, respiratory, cardiovascular, endocrine, nervous, gastrointestinal, and even reproductive systems.[2] That's essentially every part of our body.

Our hormones (primarily cortisol) are designed to support our bodies temporarily in extremely challenging and stressful events, but when they are constantly triggered, our body cannot thrive. Cortisol, which usually helps regulate our immune system, becomes overactive under chronic stress. The innate connection between our gut and brain can be damaged. Our body is thrown out of balance and begins the dangerous cycle of attacking itself. Our body's stress response is meant to support us in our most challenging moments, not to be constantly, chronically active. When we live "stressed out," "busy" lives, we aren't wearing a badge of honor; we are actually doing damage—physically, mentally, and spiritually.

The other way we see this focus on convenience in our meals play out is in the food itself. The truth is, especially when it comes to food, what is convenient is very rarely what's best. There may be a time and place for making that trade off, but it shouldn't be our pattern of life. When food is convenient, that primarily means that someone else is preparing it for you, either a restaurant or a factory. In either case, when you can't see what's actually going into your food, you give away control. When you don't have control over what is going into your body, you are doomed before you start. No one (or no company) is going to prioritize your body more than you are. There will always be competing interests when you trust others with your food.

This principle is most clearly seen in the rapid rise of over-processed foods that make up far too much of the average American's diet. We'll look more specifically at these in the next chapter, but for now what's important is recognizing that we are so drawn to over-processed foods because they are about as efficient as food can get. They include boxed cereals, granola bars, bagged potato chips, and really anything that comes in a box or bag that you don't have to worry about expiring—these "foods" are not food in reality (just check their ingredients). They are efficiency traps that turn our lust for convenience against us.

Once foods have been that over-processed, they are so far removed from the plant or animal they came from that they no longer resemble their source at all. As a consequence, they almost wholly lack the actual nutrients God designed for us to gain from them.

So, if this lust for convenience with our food is really so detrimental, why do we keep running to it? If we're honest, the productive efficiency mindset we live in, oftentimes, is simply a facade to cover our selfishness. We want to use our time how *we* want to use it. We have things to do, shows to watch, people to see. Why should we waste our time preparing a home-cooked meal? It's a misordered appetite that takes our eyes off God and puts them on ourselves. If we structure our lives so that we need to minimize something that God seems to prioritize, that should cause us to pause.

When Haley's body started failing her, it quickly became obvious how much we let convenience dictate our meal choices. We were living the typical American young professional lifestyle. Haley had a long commute into a big city, we had lots of events to attend, and people to see. Meals were squeezed in and often eaten out. When her health deteriorated and she subsequently committed to a radical change in her diet, that meant making the space to cook *all* her meals at home. We needed to make sure that everything she was putting into her body was helping her heal and we couldn't do that at a restaurant or from packaged products.

The dramatic shift from convenience-focused meals to intentional mealtimes was not easy. Early on, Haley felt isolated and over-whelmed. Her diet was so limited that she would have to cook her own meals separately from mine. It all needed to be done a certain way, with certain foods of a certain quality. She had to make sure she had enough to pack for lunch the next day (plus any snacks she would want) because she couldn't just grab something out if she was hungry. She had a supplement routine and constant appointments to manage. We were shopping at new stores and reading all the labels. We were listening to podcasts and reading books to try to absorb any helpful information we could. All the while, she was still feeling the pain of her Ulcerative Colitis. It felt like her whole life was consumed by working around her food. As her husband, I desperately wanted to help as much as I could, but I really didn't know how. It was a challenging, inconvenient time.

But you know what? God used that challenge to draw us closer as a couple and to reveal the idol of convenience in our lives. We credit that period of our marriage for teaching us how to work together as a team. I learned more of what it meant to lay down my life for my wife as Christ did for the church. Haley was able to grow in allowing me to help bear her burdens with her. And, importantly, it got easier.

As we saw the incredible results she was having, we gained confidence and motivation to continue. She was able to add more and more foods into her diet. We got better (and faster) at cooking meals as we spent more time in the kitchen. We found planning rhythms that helped us not feel overwhelmed. We learned what foods were helping her heal, so grocery trips got quicker. Eventually, when Haley was further along in the process, we even found some convenient packaged options that we could feel good about putting into our bodies. The incredible inconvenience at the beginning of her journey shaped our mindset for the latter part of her journey. Now our mealtime doesn't feel like an inconvenience. That's partially because we have that first year or so to contrast with. But it is also because we no longer see food as an inconvenience but rather as a daily reminder of God's healing provision in our lives.

This all goes to say that pursuing God's design for our food is something that is just plain impossible to do without time. You don't have to clear your entire schedule, but you do need to be willing to make some sacrifices. Remember, it's not about a set of rules. I'm not saying grabbing Chipotle in your twenty minutes between classes is inherently wrong or sinful. I'm not even saying that convenience in and of itself is bad. There are ways to make home-cooked meals more convenient yet still align with God's good design for our food. In its proper place, convenience can even make home cooking a more sustainable path forward. That may look like meal prepping for the week or a hodge-podge meal of leftovers. In Part III, we'll even discuss how to choose the highest quality processed options for when you really need them.

I'm not suggesting convenience can't be a powerful tool. What I am suggesting is that we must be cautious to not elevate convenience to a place that it doesn't deserve in our lives. Don't let a God-given desire to steward our time well become a misordered appetite masking selfishness in our hearts. Instead, let's consider if God has a purpose and design for our mealtimes.

Maybe He set them up not to hold you back but to help you flourish.

Maybe He built them in to give you a few moments of rest in a busy schedule.

Maybe He set aside time for you to thank Him for His daily provision and cast your burdens on Him.

Maybe He scheduled daily fellowship time with those you love most because He knows how much family is connected to flourishing.

Maybe, just maybe, He also prepared a path to healing for us around the table.

How can we ever realize that if our meals are hijacked by convenience?

I hope that you can begin to see mealtime not as wasted time to be reduced, but valuable time to be cherished. Ask yourself this (imperfect yet helpful) diagnostic question, *What percentage of my food comes from a box, bag, or restaurant?* Then, make a concerted effort to minimize that number. Try a week of prioritizing making fresh, home-cooked meals with the people you love most. It doesn't need to be a Michelin Star-level meal every night. It just takes simple, quality ingredients and a few dedicated minutes. Then, enjoy your reward around the table with your favorite people. Ask each other questions about your day, your faith, your highs, your lows, how God has provided, and how you are asking Him to provide again. Take a chance on something that our culture would say is a foolish waste of time, but that our God says is precious and valuable. Don't let convenience corrupt your food.

Chapter 7
Corporate Shortcuts

Now that we've considered how we can personally overemphasize convenience in our lives, let's take a look at how that misordered appetite can be played to by deceptive practices in our world. Of course, any organization, official or unofficial, is made up of individuals. Like every one of us, those individuals are sinful and therefore surrender to their own flesh's appetites at a personal level. However, when those personal pitfalls are shared among the majority, they start to take on a life of their own. Systems are shaped around deceptive practices, and we're all affected by them. These practices take advantage of our personally misordered appetites and make the path towards God's design narrower.

That's not to say that we aren't responsible for our own actions, but it is to say that we don't live in a vacuum. In fact, we all live right smack dab in the middle of a culture that tells us that money, pleasure, and time are all that matter. Often, it is too easy to nod our heads and move on. To begin to discover some of these deceptive practices of the world around us can be brutal and disheartening. But remember, this isn't the end of the story; it's just the conflict. There is a brighter, better future in God's design for food and healing in our lives.

When it comes to how we, as a Western society, have fallen short of the beautiful design that God has for our healing, money has to be at the heart of it. We'll save that topic for last. But as they say, time is money. Convenience certainly sells these days. A study published in the *American Journal of Clinical Nutrition* studied the food purchasing habits of American households from 2000 to 2012. What they found was that more than 75% of food we, as a nation, bought (measured in calories) was at least moderately processed. What's more amazing is that more than 60% of our calories are *highly* processed (which they define as "multi-ingredient industrially formulated mixtures").[1]

Read that again. The significant majority of the food we buy is an "industrially formulated mixture." The image in your head should be examples like chicken nuggets, breakfast cereal, chips, pretzels, cookies, candy, etc. If you buy it in a box or bag and it's ready-to-eat, then it likely fits in this category. What's fascinating is those stats were steady trends across the 12-year period of the study. These foods have become our norm.

Talk about a monopoly on a market! Processed foods rule the day. And the corporations that sell them to us know that all too well. They get the best of both worlds: over-processing the foods creates a product that never goes bad and is so unnaturally appetizing that we can't get enough. That model essentially prints money. Just ask a company like PepsiCo, whose whole business is highly processed foods and beverages (excluding bottled water). PepsiCo alone owns *twenty-two* unique food and beverage brands that make at least a billion dollars annually (e.g. Fritos, Tostitos, Quaker, and Mountain Dew).[2] Twenty-two! Large food companies have figured out the magic formula and they're sticking to it. It's called convenience. Our culture sells us the lie that we need to be so busy that convenient, over-processed food is our only option. However, not only is that food directly deteriorating our health, but the stress levels of an overstuffed life itself are ripping us apart from the inside. We have bought into the message from the propaganda machine, but it isn't the path to life.

Processing a food, in and of itself, isn't always bad. Technically, freezing, pickling, and fermenting are all forms of processing a food. Processing just means transforming a food from its untouched form to something else. Simply put, it's going through a process. Many of these simple processing techniques have been around for most of human history and can even add healing potential to our foods. For example, fermenting a food adds beneficial probiotics to it, and sprouting grains makes them much more digestible.

However, when processing the food gets to the point where the result no longer resembles its origin, we need to question the value of that convenience against the value of its nutrition. Traditional processes, such as pickling, use a combination of simple ingredients (e.g. salt and water) and time. These processes don't change the basic complexion of the food. In contrast, over-processing aims to "promote shelf stability, preserve texture, and increase palatability."[3] It combines harsh chemicals, intense heat, and artificial additives to convert the original ingredients into something entirely different. These shortcuts are irresistible to these massive food producers because their food will last forever, taste great, and print money.

So, what's so wrong with our beloved multi-ingredient industrially formulated mixtures, anyway? The problem is at least three-pronged. First, the discord between the low effort to acquire these products and the high pleasure we receive from consuming them is both psychologically and physiologically destructive (more on this next chapter). The pleasure of a food that used to take hours or even days to prepare can now be generated in a matter of seconds. Secondly, they are what some have labeled "hyper-palatable." Basically, this means that they are unnaturally desirable. This is due in part to the fact that they are essentially pre-chewed for us by the ultra-processing they go through, continuing to confuse our internal reward system. Finally, and perhaps most obviously, the ingredients that make up our "multi-ingredient industrially formulated mixtures" are often, well, industrial. Since the end product looks and tastes amazing, and we don't get any view into the process, companies are free to cut any corners they'd like.

"Our breakfast cereal looks dull? Let's add some Red #3 [artificial food dye made from petroleum] to spice things up!"

"The customers don't like stirring their peanut butter? They won't mind a touch of hydrogenated canola oil [hidden trans fat] to keep it spreadable!"

"Our ice cream isn't quite creamy enough? Let's add carrageenan [an emulsifier linked to inflammation and cancer] to smooth that out!"

The ends justify the means for these corporations. They fall into the convenience trap like any one of us would, but when these major food producers cut corners, the scale of the destruction is much wider. Our food supply ends up over-processed and overstuffed with ugly additives that we would never use in our own kitchens.

The truth is that most highly processed foods have simply been stripped of the vitamins, minerals, enzymes, and beneficial bacteria that make them part of God's healing design for us. In fact, one study showed that ultra-processed foods have less than half of the micronutrients of their natural counterparts. [4] If you think about it, everything that we were designed to eat was alive at some point. It's that *living* aspect of food that contributes to our healing. It's what supports the balance of our gut microbiome, which in turn helps us flourish. On the other hand, the more we strip food of its natural beauty, the more *dead* it becomes. Oftentimes, it's so dead that it hurts us more than it helps.

The over-processing of food is the most obvious example of the deceptive practices that food producers use to maximize their convenience over our health, but it is really just the end product of the so-called optimized industrial food industry. As the *Journal of Hunger and Environmental Nutrition* explains, this industrialization includes the rise in new farming technologies, globalization, government subsidies, and crop specialization.[5] Those things all sound perfectly harmless, even helpful on the surface, but they have major consequences on the quality of our food and our body's healing power.

New farming technologies can include neutral or positive innovations like tractors and irrigation, but they can also include entirely harmful changes, such as genetically modified organisms (also known as GMOs) and pesticides. These technologies increase productivity of your typical industrial farm, ultimately allowing for massive consolidation of farming. Consolidation (within an ever more global society) plus the technology to preserve and ship crops anywhere in the world has allowed for a relative few to gain a disproportionately large level of power in the agricultural world. This influence leads to government policies that only help keep this process "optimized" for those in power. Government policies subsidize certain crops (primarily corn and soy), incentivizing massive farms to focus primarily on these crops. That means they aren't growing a diversity of plants and likely aren't raising livestock at all. Crops aren't being rotated in those fields, which depletes the nutrients in the soil. Insects feast on the unchanging fuel source, and the natural fertilizer of animal manure is nowhere to be found on the farm. These so-called optimizations feed the nasty cycle of needing more and more synthetic chemical fertilizers and pesticides, which all end up on our food and in our gut.

All of these shortcuts are great for the producers but ruinous for our food supply. By the time our food reaches our plates, it's been modified, sprayed, preserved, shipped, and stored. These practices are as deceptive as they come. They are convenient for those gaining from them, but the consumer is the one who pays the price. For example, according to the Center for Food Safety, GMOs may potentially be connected to nutrient loss, suppression of our immune systems, and even cancer.[6] When we acknowledge that God designed our food to be our healing fuel, we should question practices that dramatically reduce their healing potential, especially in the name of corporate shortcuts.

Convenience—or its sister, efficiency—plays a role in so many cultural practices. Convenience is a tsunami of pressure whose rip tide will drown you if you aren't careful. This is true of our farm system and it's true in our healthcare system. If we have a headache, we pop an ibuprofen. If our mental health is failing, we take an antidepressant. If our immune system is failing us, we take the injection. If the doctors can't figure out the issue, we take an antibiotic. There's a pill for everything (this extends to the health world with quick-fix-promising supplements, too). About **66%** of Americans are on a prescription drug and most of the rest use some sort of over-the-counter drug.[7] I'm sure most doctors have the best of intentions, but for whatever reason, they tend to take the most convenient path. Ironically, one of the primary reasons they do this is the long line of people in their waiting room whose eating habits have left them in shambles.

The issue with accepting the seemingly convenient path by blindly accepting pharmaceuticals is that it's often just a band-aid, and there are always side effects. There are the more obvious side effects that we laugh about because half of every drug commercial is spent blabbing about them—things like higher risk of certain cancers or blood clots. But there are also the more subtle side effects, the ones that come from a constant exposure to synthetic, inorganic substances. Effects including imbalance and inflammation slowly but surely lead to disastrous results. We may be worried about efficiency, but chronic disease garners no such concern. It keeps trucking along, little by little, until it becomes a full-blown crisis. While we get our quick fix from our present symptoms, we ignore the slow but steady outcomes we're being led towards. Our battle is far too often against our symptoms, which can be suppressed (for a time), instead of the root cause, which silently lingers in the background. We are fighting a losing battle because we fight consistency with convenience.

True healing takes time. Yes, there is a time and place for Western medicine. I don't deny that. However, the way we eat, drink, sleep, de-stress, and detox can heal you. The way we live matters. It's a simple but slow truth. The grocery store, the global supply chain, and the hospital all have their own prerogatives, which are all measured in a quarterly earnings statement.

They can't afford to look long-term.

You can't afford not to.

You will live in your body for the rest of your life. No one else will rediscover God's ancient design for you; it's something you need to do on your own. Then, you have to fight to live in that flourishing path. It doesn't come by way of a quick fix. It is not a path of instant gratification. It may take a radical lifestyle change that makes you uncomfortable and slows your pace of life. But it can also set you free in a way that you didn't know possible. Convenience is a cheap substitute for God's good, healing design.

Chapter 8
Tantalizing Taste

Taste. It's always one of the essential categories evaluated in any competition cooking show. And rightfully so. I mean, what would food be without flavor? Imagine for a moment that food didn't taste like anything. What if food was simply chunks of matter that we ingested to stay alive? How much different would our lives be? No need to seek out Saturday night reservations at the new restaurant in town. No sense of the sweet bite of the summer's first peach. Life would be a lot less fun, truly. Taste is without a doubt a gift from God. However, when the good desire for a delicious taste becomes the ultimate purpose of our food, it becomes a misordered appetite that can wreak havoc in our lives.

Remember, we take after our first parents, Adam and Eve. They saw the forbidden fruit as a "delight to the eyes." That fruit, whatever it was, must've looked pretty darn tasty. It must've looked like a sleeve of Oreos or a slice of cheesecake or something. Seriously, what kind of fruit looked so good that they were willing to break the one rule that God had given them? They fell prey to their misordered appetite, and that is exactly what the typical American consumer does, too. Eve said, "It looks good, it must be good," and we've followed her footsteps just the same.

Look, God certainly wants us to enjoy the beautiful taste of His food. Jesus calls His followers the "salt of the earth" in Matthew 5:13. At least part of that illustration must be in regards to the mighty flavor of salt. In Psalm 34:8, the psalmist even uses the metaphor of taste to give a picture of just how enjoyable it is to know God and take refuge in Him: "Taste and see that the Lord is good!" When Jesus used the metaphor of the fattened calf in the story of the prodigal son (Luke 15:23), it was because everyone would've known how great that steak would have tasted! More generally, God is the creator of life. He wants us to enjoy that life and ultimately to enjoy Him. That includes many wonderful tastes that He perfectly designed. I can only imagine the stunning flavor of the fruit of the (permitted) trees of the Garden of Eden. God often uses His creation and our senses to reveal something of Himself to us, and taste is no exception. It can be a nearly spiritual experience to enjoy God's good gift to us in the form of food. That experience helps us to know and enjoy the God who designed our food and our ability to taste it.

So, I am certainly not trying to argue that we shouldn't eat food that tastes good. In fact, I would say that most everything Haley and I eat is delicious! At the same time, I would suggest that most of us have lost the ability to *know* what tastes good.

Let me explain.

Our palates have been cauterized by the lab-designed flavor vehicle we call "food" today. Real, from-the-ground foods taste bland or even bad to many of us. Whether it's an aversion to trying new things, an addiction to over-processed flavor bombs, or simply poorly prepared "healthy" foods that leave a bad taste in our mouth (literally), we are stuck. We're stuck in a place where the only things that taste good to us are designed not by God, but by a lab. Plants and animals were the original food. That's what they were designed for. If we "don't like" them, I think it says more about us than it does about the food.

If I asked you what part of tasty foods are bad for you, I bet you would say sugar, fat, or both. In a sense, you'd be right. But in another, not so much. What I mean is that sugar and fat aren't inherently evil. They're really not. God made them both and they each have a purpose for us. They have a way to be enjoyed that is right and good.

As we've often done throughout this book, we can look back at how our ancestors lived as a helpful comparison. For most of human existence, sugar was primarily found in fruits. Fruit was the original sweet treat! Most fruits' sugar content would peak when it was perfectly ripe. As various fruits ripened throughout the year, our ancestors would have a small, steady, seasonal diet of naturally occurring sugars. Fruit would give our ancestors a perfect energy boost. God designed our food, even sugar, to taste the best when it was the best for us.

When it comes to fat, that's typically something we try not to *be* and therefore try not to *eat*, right? Well, again, God designed fat with a purpose in mind. At its best, fat stores energy, helps absorb nutrients, and even powers our brain.[1] Our ancestors would have rejoiced at the chance to partake of a particularly fatty meal because it offered their body a resilient strength. They would've mostly eaten fats in traditional fashions like olives, butter, nuts, fish, lamb, beef, and other animals. These natural fats had positive—not negative—effects on their bodies, and they tasted great, too! God has a plan for all of His creation, remember?

So, if sugar and fat taste great and were designed to be good for us, what went wrong? Our appetites have been misordered so that the taste itself is the most important consideration when choosing our sustenance. In the words of Philippians 3:19, our god is our belly. We live in a world that tells us that we should have what we want, when we want it. That we should live our best life. A world of "you deserve it, go take it." Those deceptive ideas have engulfed our diets in a dark shadow. The toxic combination of industrialized food and a culture of self-actualization has turned us into junk food junkies simply because it tastes good.

Another way to think about this idea is that our internal reward system is broken. Our ancestors wanted sugar and fat as much as we do. That innate signal isn't wrong; it's actually built in. The difference is that our ancestors put their blood, sweat, and tears into cultivating sweet and fatty delicacies. When our ancestors finally were able to enjoy summer strawberries or a ribeye, it was because they had put in the work of cultivating a garden or raising livestock. Then, after that hard work, they reaped the delicious benefits. This system acted to motivate them to continue the hard work of life even when it was uncomfortable. They would be rewarded in due time.

That same reward system exists in our brains today. Our brains are full of receptors for chemicals like dopamine which regulate this natural reward system. Basically, a boost in dopamine is experienced as a reward for something good happening. Foods with high sugar and fat contents draw out these dopamine hits in our brain. That worked for our ancestors, but the problem is that in today's world, we do nearly zero work for the unnaturally potent rewards of ultra-processed versions of sugar and fat. When we feel the dopamine effect (say from a bag of Doritos), our brains assume we must've done something right. It tells us that we should do that again. And again. And again. In fact, the consistent dopamine hits from a high sugar diet decreases our brain's ability to experience it at all.[2] This forces us to need more and more for the same euphoria. Since ultra-processed foods are so readily available, getting more isn't an issue. We can have whatever we want, whenever we want it, with no work necessary. It's a vicious cycle leading to what essentially becomes an addiction to unnatural taste.

The dawn of over-processed foods packed with sugar was only about a hundred years ago. Since then, anyone could observe that our collective health quickly deteriorated. In particular, we were gaining lots of weight. We were getting fatter, and it wasn't long until we were told to blame fat itself, especially saturated fats, which are mostly found in animal-based products like butter or beef (something that many studies have since debunked—more on this in Part III).

Since we certainly didn't lose our taste for fats when we were told they were "bad for us," this opened the door for a new world of so-called "heart healthy" fats made from "vegetables." Unfortunately, the vast majority of "vegetable oils" are highly refined, industrial products that force fat from cheap sources (e.g. seeds from crops like soybeans, corn, canola, etc.). Mankind couldn't even squeeze oil out of most of these seeds until the industrial revolution![3] The seed-based oil extraction process requires a chemical solvent called hexane which is a known neurotoxin.[4] In some cases, the oils themselves are actually toxic before they're ultra-refined and deodorized. But that didn't stop corporations from putting them in essentially every form of over-processed food. They hide in plain sight.

These cheap, seed-based oils don't satisfy us the way that traditional, unprocessed fats do, so the industrial food system found a work-around with (you guessed it) more chemical processing techniques. The process is called hydrogenation and it is a chemical reaction that forces seed-based oils to act like animal fats by changing their chemistry to stay solid at room temperature. This creates trans fat (trans means that the fat has changed form). Trans fat is considered the most detrimental form of fat, yet it is so prevalent in our pre-packaged, shelf-stable foods. In fact, the synthetic version of trans fat was determined to be so bad for us that the FDA banned it in 2015. Though this was progress, it has not eliminated over-processed, trans fats from our diets.

Perhaps the most damaging part of this fat swap was how it played to our misordered appetite for taste over everything. Because these new-fangled seed-based oils just didn't taste the same as the traditional, unprocessed fats our ancestors lived on, we weren't satisfied with them. They weren't the same. So, what did big food producers do? They packed our food full of the other ancient reward-system stimulator: sugar.

The ancient diet would not have included significant sugar consumption. When our ancestors did enjoy sugar, it would come alongside the fruit's fiber to help metabolize it evenly. Now our sugar has been isolated, concentrated, and added to everything. Even as recently as the late 1700s, the average American only ate around six pounds of sugar per year. That number in 2017? One hundred thirty pounds per year.[5]

One hundred thirty.

That number should floor you. We eat more sugar in a month than someone in the 1700s ate in a year. What's perhaps even crazier, is that that number is down from its peak (around 1999). But in today's world, sugar is hiding everywhere. While refined cane sugar consumption has decreased substantially since 1970, corn-based sweeteners (like high fructose corn syrup) have increased to an even greater degree in that time.[6] We are (and I mean this in the truest sense) addicted to the stuff; we cannot stop ourselves. God designed sugar to be a sweet treat, a sign of ripeness, and even a burst of energy. We now crave it as a necessity of life. Unfortunately, food producers, whose primary drive is to sell more food, have used our God-given desire for tasty food against us in four easy steps:

Step 1: Over-processed seed-based oils keep their products cheap.

Step 2: Isolated, concentrated sugar masks the unsatisfying bland oil and simultaneously gives our brain a hit of dopamine.

Step 3: We can access it all without having to lift a finger.

Step 4: Our innate reward system thinks we did something right, triggering us to want more and more until we're hooked.

This all combined to radicalize our taste buds. The University of Michigan studied this phenomenon and discovered that a high sugar diet may reduce the number of "cells required to detect sweet, bitter, and umami" flavors, plus the nerve response to sugar was reduced by almost 50%.[7] Basically, the more sugar we eat, the less it satisfies, and the more muted our other taste senses become.

We have misordered our natural, good appetite for tasty food to make it king and, in the process, have lost the ability to enjoy true food. Our world has redefined taste in an unnatural way. What's devastating about this is that we also lose some of our ability to be inspired and awestruck by what our good God has given us. While it is certainly possible to praise God for the enjoyment of over-processed food, it seems to me that we are much more likely to do so with food directly designed by God, since we can see His beautiful creativity so clearly. Honestly, when was the last time a Snickers made you give praise to God? Or an Oreo made you shout forth thanksgiving? If the food we eat is designed by man, then we're more likely to thank man. If it's designed by God, then we're more likely to thank God!

God wants us to enjoy Him, and one of the spectacular ways we get to do that is by enjoying His food. He's the Father who serves the delicious fattened calf when the prodigal son returns, after all! We lose at least some of our spiritual ability to "taste and see that the

Lord is good" if our physical ability to taste His good food has been seared. Trust me, God's food is delicious! Although, it might not start that way for you. It may, in fact, be a shock to your system. It may take a self-reflective evaluation of your reward system. It might take some serious taste bud recalibration. But there is real hope for change. In fact, that same University of Michigan study discovered that the effects of the high sugar diet on taste buds are reversible. God designed even our taste buds to heal.

The early stages of Haley's healing journey weren't the epitome of flavor. She ate a lot of boiled chicken, hard-boiled eggs, and steamed carrots. She didn't even use spices at the very beginning. Things were pretty bland. Plus, Haley has always been a dessert lover. Cutting out all refined sugar was not easy. No Ghirardelli brownies or Ben & Jerry's. But, again, God showed Himself. The reduced refined sugar may have been the single most impactful part of her healing journey. Her body was able to reduce inflammation, reset, and rejuvenate.

It was worth it to sacrifice flavor (temporarily) for healing. Even then, we found simple treats to enjoy. We experienced firsthand the radical change your taste buds can experience. In contrast to no sugar, even simple options like homemade applesauce or baked fruit tasted extraordinary! Of course, over time, we've expanded the dessert menu (think: homemade fudge and ice cream) while focusing on using natural sugars and whole foods.

As for non-dessert food, as Haley added more and more foods back into her diet, we experimented with options we'd never eaten before. We tried new things like spaghetti squash, fennel, bok choy, dates, figs, chia seeds, lamb, turmeric, and mushrooms. We found that oftentimes we truly enjoyed things we initially thought we wouldn't. We weren't just saying "No" to all the pizza, cake, and cookies we'd eaten our whole lives. We were saying "Yes" to a new world of exploration of all the real food we'd been missing! Today, we don't feel deprived of flavor in the least. On the contrary, we love getting to explore all the brilliantly designed, multi-faceted flavors that God perfectly placed in His food. They are far better than the one-note sweetness that fills much of our engineered foods today.

Over time, we learned that it isn't about self-denial for self-denial's sake; rather, it's about trusting that God gave us all we need to be satisfied. The original, true food is what we were built to eat and enjoy. It was designed by a good God who gives good gifts. If you believe in this God, it makes sense to believe that He gives us food that we can and should enjoy. But don't misorder your appetites to put taste as your primary pursuit because we ultimately enjoy food to enjoy the God who made it.

Chapter 9
The Taste Pitch

We talked in the last chapter about how we can idolize taste in our Western culture. While we certainly have personal responsibility for our food choices, we also discussed how the practices of large food producers have led us to that astounding overconsumption of refined sugars and over-processed fats. That is one side of the taste story. The other side is the corporate sales pitch that has been set up to sell flavor over everything.

The pitch is two-sided. First (and more obviously), we are being sold a product. Whether it's Oreos, Pizza Hut, Reese's Cups, Gatorade, or whatever, food marketing is almost constantly in front of our faces. According to the *International Journal of Behavioral Nutrition and Physical Activity*, "the US Food System is the second largest advertiser in the American economy."[1] The largest categories of food advertising included breakfast cereals, candy/gum, soft drinks, and snacks. Each of these fit in the over-processed category. Another study estimated that children are exposed to marketing for "non-core" or not recommended food or drink products 27.3 times per day.[2] The advertising of many of these brands are brightly colored, meant to draw your eye and trick your brain to want that product.

The point is that billions and billions of dollars are spent every year to get you (or your kids) to buy their product. Once you buy it, well, that's all she wrote. The refined sugars and over-processed fats do their thing, releasing that hit of dopamine to our brains each time we eat them. This is even more powerful when artificial sweeteners are used to lower caloric intake because our bodies expect and crave those calories from the sweet flavor.[3] Companies are quite literally making us feel a momentary high, which forms borderline obsessive thoughts around their products.

These processed, taste-forward foods are full of engineered additives that are only developed to taste or look good. At best, these additives provide no health benefits, but more likely they are detrimental. These additives are things like artificial flavors, food dyes, high fructose corn syrup, diacetyl, brominated vegetable oil, titanium dioxide, and potassium bromate (each of which have their own documented health risks).[4]

However, the biggest culprit of them all is one of the most common ingredients you'll see on food labels from Walmart to Whole Foods: "natural flavors." Now, this might sound innocent at first, but it is actually a blanket term that could mean just about anything. Genetically modified ingredients are not even excluded from being labeled "natural flavors." The formulation of the flavors themselves is barely regulated. Dr. Luke Grocholl, a regulatory affairs expert at a company that (among other things) works on gene editing, mRNA development, and "flavor and fragrance formulation" says this:

"There is little restriction on manufacturing processes in declaring flavors as natural. For example, isolation of natural flavors through chemical transformation by inorganic catalysts meets the US natural flavor requirement. As an example, 2-methyl-2-pentenoic acid (FEMA# 2923) manufacturing by the base-catalyzed condensation of propionaldehyde isolated from fusel oil is considered natural. In this case, the raw material (fusel oil) is considered a natural raw material since it is the by-product of alcohol fermentation. The intermediate is isolated by distillation, a physical process, then undergoes chemical transformation via a catalyst, followed by oxidation by heating in air, and finally further purification by distillation."[5]

Does any of that sound "natural" to you? You may be wondering why these companies would go through all that trouble. The answer is quite simple: a concentrated and distinctly *un*natural flavor is so potent that it distorts our taste buds so that only *their* flavor satisfies us. In other words, we have to buy more. And the competitors' products, let alone actual real food, aren't good enough.

These chemicals are thrown into our foods without thought of how they might affect our long-term health. Many of them are never studied at all, let alone for long-term exposure or their interaction with the thousands of other chemicals the average consumer is exposed to on a daily basis. How are these additives affecting our immune systems? our hormones? our microbiome? We simply don't know. We are chronically, and mostly unknowingly, exposed to these chemicals and that must have a profound effect on our bodies' ability to heal and flourish.

The other side of the processed food industry's taste pitch is much more subtle, but I think much more damaging. Children may be susceptible to the colorful marketing ploys trying to sell candy or cereals, but we adults are too smart for that to influence us, right? Well, the sales pitch matures with us. It's a faux grassroots campaign that gains traction from word-of-mouth. And it's a smear campaign. We're sold the lie that nutritious eating is tasteless eating.

And that it's too hard.

And that it's inconvenient.

And that it's a fad.

And that it's expensive.

And that you'll miss out.

And that you'll never be satisfied.

This has probably never been more clearly illustrated than by KFC's award-winning 2017 "Dirty Louisiana" ad campaign. KFC realized that more and more people were trying to eat healthier at the same time they were trying to release their self-proclaimed "most indulgent burger." The creators of this ad campaign had an unashamed message: "Challenge the joylessness of 'clean eating' with the indulgent taste of the Dirty Louisiana."

The actual campaign culminated in the creation of a fake food blogger's "collaboration" with KFC to create the "Clean Eating Burger." The key characteristics of this burger were bland taste, hard-to-find ingredients, and general pretentiousness. At the end of the ad, the tiny, white, flavorless "Clean Eating Burger" is destroyed by the giant, colorful, overflowing "Dirty Louisiana." Finally, a narrator seals the deal by saying, "Nothing satisfies like a Dirty Louisiana." And you know what? "The Dirty Louisiana became one of KFC's best-selling LTOs (Limited Time Offers) of the last 5 years, selling out of 70% of stores nationally within 3 weeks and surpassing the sales mix target by 39%."[6]

Most companies aren't nearly that overt, but they all use those same tactics. We've been trained to think that it's only the health nuts that can actually maintain that lifestyle—and even when they do, they're depriving themselves of the good stuff. They're missing out on all their favorite foods. They don't actually *like* it. They aren't satisfied. They are joyless.

Folks, this is a lie.

It's the lie being told to the 4-year-old seeing ads for Coco Crisps and Chips Ahoy 27.3 times a day. That same lie convinces the 24-year-old that they don't like the taste of green beans. Or the 43-year-old to never try butternut squash. Or the 67-year-old to live off frozen pizzas and take out.

The truth is our bodies were meant to love the taste of the food that God created for us. God designed the food in the Garden of Eden to be "pleasant to the sight and good for food" (Genesis 2:9). Along with the nutrition inherent in God's original food, there was some "pleasant" quality about it, too. It wasn't God's plan that for millennia humankind would suffer through tasteless, unsatisfying meals until one day someone in the 20th century invented corn syrup. On the contrary, the truth is that food, the way God made it, tastes amazing. I'm talking mind-blowing, out-of-this-world, can't-believe-I-used-to-say-I-didn't-like-this amazing. It is utterly satisfying.

KFC (and the processed, taste-forward food industry it represents) wants you to believe you need them to find joy, but our God has given us everything we need to find joy in Him and in His design.

I desperately want you to experience this truth, but the only way that is possible is if you disentangle from the great American sales pitch and try it for yourself. When I say try, I don't mean doing a 30-day diet or microwaving broccoli one night this week. I mean commit to changing habits and lifestyles, persevering when it seems like things won't change. If we're changing decades of habits to move in the right direction, it's not going to be easy, but it is going to be worth it.

Remember, food was never, primarily, about taste. We've idolized this one aspect of it because it's what our senses experience most. It elicits quick, immediate feedback from our bodies. Our brains and our stomachs want more. But that is not the *primary* purpose for which God gave us food. Yes, He gave us the incredible gift of our sense of taste. And absolutely, He wants us to enjoy the spectacular flavors that *He* designed. I hope that you do. But as far back as Genesis 1, God was connecting the idea of what we eat to our flourishing. When we eat only to please our taste buds, we misorder our appetite for pleasure over purpose. Food is the fuel for the healing engine of our God-designed bodies. It should be our first step towards flourishing in a toxic world. It should help us, not hurt us. *And* it can taste great doing it.

Chapter 10
Counting the Costs

Is there any topic in the world that gets emotions and conflict going the way money does? Most people would rather talk to a stranger about religion and politics than about their money. But money reaches every area of our lives. You probably think about it more than just about anything else in your life. In fact, a 2015 poll found that at least 25% of Americans say that it is the thing they think about most on a daily basis, more than their love life, health, politics, and on par with their day job.[1] For that matter, most people wouldn't think about their day job nearly as much if it wasn't their primary source of money.

Money can be an intense stressor in our lives, yet it very rarely provides any sort of joy, in and of itself. Sure, you can feel relief when the paycheck comes in or you can buy something that makes you smile, but money itself almost always brings stress and conflict. The problem is that we give money too inflated a role in our lives. Yes, money has value and purpose, but we tend to think that it means far more than it truly does. This is true of American society, maybe more than most, but it is also a timeless truth, one that even the biblical authors had to consider. For example, the author of Ecclesiastes writes:

> "Wisdom and money can get you almost anything, but only wisdom can save your life."
>
> ECCLESIASTES 7:12 (NLT)

The author gives a sober value to money—it can be helpful. However, he also says that we are too quick to conflate wisdom and money. We see wealth and assume wisdom. But this verse points out the folly in that thought process. Though money does offer us some provision, true wisdom is what has the power to preserve our lives. Let's also look at just a little of what Jesus had to say about this topic (He says a whole lot more, too!):

> "And Jesus said to his disciples, 'Truly, I say to you, only with difficulty will a rich person enter the kingdom of heaven. Again I tell you, it is easier for a camel to go through the eye of a needle than for a rich person to enter the kingdom of God.' When the disciples heard this, they were greatly astonished, saying, 'Who then can be saved?'"
>
> MATTHEW 19:23-25

Jesus directly combats the idea that wealth has some deeper meaning about worth or wisdom. In fact, He makes it quite clear that more money makes true wisdom significantly harder to obtain. The disciples' response is a really honest, though misguided one—and that is what makes it so relatable; we are prone to the same thought! The disciples thought, "Goodness, if the guy who has his affairs in order and seems to have this whole life thing under control can't make it into the kingdom of heaven, who can?!" They linked worldly wealth with wisdom.

Money makes for a poor master, though we are quick to give it that role—especially when the world starts to praise us for our wealth. We lose sight of God's true wisdom, namely, the Gospel, which says that we are morally and spiritually bankrupt, but we can become heirs of the Most High God with heavenly riches unfathomable through the free gift of grace that is the cross of Christ.

Eve's third misordered appetite in the garden was that the forbidden fruit seemed desirable to make her wise. She saw something God created and was deceived into thinking that it could offer her something that the Creator Himself couldn't. Isn't that the essence of any so-called wisdom that is not from God Himself? Isn't that often the essence of our twisted relationship with money? We far too often believe this created thing can offer us something that the Creator can't. This is not wisdom; it is a misordered appetite which leads to death.

Can we make enough, save enough, spend enough, invest enough, or maybe even give enough to gain what we want? Even if your hope is in the American dream, the answer is "No." But if your hope is in the Kingdom of Heaven, it's a resounding "Absolutely not!" Don't buy the world's greatest lie, forsaking God's good design to run full steam ahead towards the false wisdom of this world called the dollar.

I hear what you're thinking right now, "Great lesson, Alex, but I thought this book was about food." You're right! So how does this all relate back to the topic at hand? Well, food costs money. Real food costs more than fake food. This is clearly a barrier to many people who agree in theory with what we've discussed thus far in this book, but they aren't ready to commit to putting it into practice. We see the insanely low prices of cheap, fake foods and we can convince ourselves that buying them is actually a wise decision. As comedian Jim Gaffigan once joked about the McDonald's dollar menu, "I don't want to lose money on this deal!"[2] It's funny, because it's true. That's exactly how we're prone to think. In the name of frugality, we run to poor options even if we know they aren't what our body needs to thrive. We end up "buying" the marketing of the deal. We convince ourselves that the economics of it are more important than the nutrition of it.

I get it. Everyone is in a different place with their bank account. Some of us have no choice but to live frugally, and there's nothing wrong with that; in fact, there is a lot right with being thoughtful about where to spend money. Just don't convince yourself that simply because you are frugal, money is not your master. The protection of money at the cost of living in God's design for your body is just as enslaving as an addiction to spending.

You don't have to be rich to live in a healing way, but you do need to make sacrifices. It's the *love* of money that is the root of all kinds of evil. No matter how much of it you have (or don't), we can all love money too much. When we love it, we idolize it. When we idolize it, we crave it. And when we crave it, we don't mind missing out on things we know to be good for our flourishing for the sake of our wallet. Let's flip that mindset. Let's trash asking *"How can I save a buck by the way I eat?"* and replace it with *"How can I glorify God by the way I eat?"*

One of the most powerful tools in our toolbox is our *mindset* about food costs. Firstly, remember that organic, whole foods were the way of essentially all of our ancestors. Though our knock-off food may be cheap, it would also be unrecognizable for most of human history. This is helpful to remind us that most of the inexpensive food we buy isn't really food in the first place. It's an industrial product designed to make money, not help us flourish. Food is the energy for all of life. Do we really want to be shopping in the bargain bin for something so important?

We're led to believe if we want to eat "healthy" it has to be expensive. Flip that narrative on its head. Instead, keep in mind that fake food is suspiciously cheap (more on this next chapter). Yes, if you replace your box of Oreos with "healthy" pre-packaged sandwich cookies, you are going to pay significantly more. But if you are replacing boxed, bagged, and restaurant food with seasonal, whole, home-cooked foods, there are cost-effective ways to eat well (we'll look more at some practical ways to make healing living a possibility on a budget in Part III of this book).

Another vital mindset change is to count the costs of the food you're eating. Don't just count the cost in dollars. Consider that, yes, but think about the bigger picture and the longer term, too.

Count the costs in inflammation and imbalance.

Count the costs in fatigue and depression.

Count the costs in doctor's appointments and insurance deductibles.

Count the cost in stress from a diagnosis and fear of the unknown.

Count the costs in constant colds and chronic disease.

Count the costs in sick days and years to recovery.

Eating primarily to save money has its costs. Maybe you haven't felt them yet, but when it comes to food, the principle of "pay me now or pay me later" applies. You may think you can get away with saving a few dollars now, but cheap, fake food leads to the compounding of chronic inflammation that leads to chronic disease (like we talked about in Part I). If you wait until you need the care of Western medicine, you'll start counting the costs a lot differently. I implore you to start investing in the best preventative medicine there is: real food.

Unfortunately, earlier in our lives, Haley and I didn't count the true costs of the food we were eating. It never even crossed our minds! We were simply living our normal American lives, never questioning if the food we were eating was poisoning us. Obviously, for Haley, this reached the point that her normal American diet led to chronic inflammation, which turned into Ulcerative Colitis. That led to years of fatigue, unhealthy weight loss, painful bowel movements, and not feeling like herself. It led to what felt like constant doctor's appointments that only seemed to suck hope away instead of offering it. It led to a feeling of unimaginable stress, confusion, and tears. It led to a years-long battle to remission, even after changing her diet in a radical way. I can tell you one thing for sure, we no longer see real food as simply "expensive", because we've been forced to count the true costs. If we could go back to before she was diagnosed, we would gladly spend a little extra money if we knew we could prevent all that she went through. I hope you never have to experience what Haley did. I hope that by counting the costs before you're forced to, you can avoid those struggles before you ever even face them.

The price of food is far too often used as an excuse not to pursue a healing lifestyle. However, like most things, it is a matter of priority. You will end up spending money one way or the other. What are you spending it on? Did you just upgrade your iPhone, but you won't upgrade to organic? Did you buy a PlayStation, but you won't buy a probiotic? Did you pay for Grubhub, but you won't pay for grass-fed beef? I urge you to at least start thinking about these things. Start questioning your spending habits. Don't let yourself use the blanket excuse of "it's too expensive" without really considering it.

There are ways to live a nourishing, God-glorifying lifestyle for any budget. The question is, *Do you want to?* Or will you let the love of money be the root of another kind of evil: neglecting the most astounding of God's creations—your body. Money and how we spend it is clearly an important topic to God. A significant portion of your budget goes to food each month. On average, Americans spend 11.3% of their income on food. Even the lowest income American households spend nearly $5,000 on food annually.[3] Money and food are intertwined whether we like it or not. But maybe you've simply never considered how love of money may be substantially affecting your body's ability to heal itself in God's good design. Or perhaps you've let money be the excuse that has prevented the healing you know you need.

Wherever you are right now, I encourage you to commit to taking the next small step in prioritizing God's design for food and healing in your budget. It doesn't need to be all at once. Consistent, small habits turn into bigger lifestyle changes. Maybe take some of the suggestions we'll get into in Part III and rank them by your own personal priority, then commit to making room in the budget for the top two or three items. Consider incorporating some of the many inexpensive or free ways to walk in God's design for healing such as moving your body, getting morning sunlight, or lowering stress levels (again, more on these in Part III).

You can be rich and not live in God's design (Jesus made that clear). So, if money is your excuse for not walking in that design now, be warned: it doesn't get any easier. Take some time to consider how you can steward your finances in a way that will steward your *body* to the glory of God a little better. In the long run, it'll pay you back in dividends!

Chapter 11
Corporate Cost-Cutting

We'll end Part II with what is probably the most obvious sin pattern across our Western society and maybe human nature as a whole: profit at all costs. If you live in America, capitalism amounts to the American dream. It promises never-ending possibilities for the future—the chance for a better life for those who have only known poverty. In order to achieve those positive outcomes, though, capitalism also—unashamedly—makes profit the great equalizer. It doesn't matter who you are, what you look like, or where you came from, if you can make a buck in America, our culture says you're worth something. It may not always be pretty, but at least it's a transparent strategy: minimize expenses, maximize revenue. At all costs.

But there are costs. Serious, even fatal costs. We can count costs in dollars, but there are so many other costs to consider, one of which is our body's God-given, healing design. The inherent, even celebrated greed on a cultural scale has led to some incredibly (and knowingly) dangerous decisions being made about our food supply.

We'll look at a few examples of this playing out but let me warn you that we are only just scratching the surface. Food comes from farms, right? Well, yes, technically, but the farm you're probably picturing in your head with the big red barn is not where most of it comes from. Most of our food comes from large, industrial farms that look more like factories than fields. In fact, large farms (greater than 1,000 acres) account for only 5.6% of all U.S. farms, yet they control 53.7% of all farmland—and that was in 2011.[1] That number is likely to be much higher today and only continue to grow. It's a corporate consolidation that we see in all major industries, but since there are so many middlemen between the Big Agriculture industry (otherwise known as Big Ag) and the end-user (otherwise known as you and me), we ignore it.

So, what are the downsides to this consolidation? Big Ag, as with all "Big" industries, mainly (only?) look at the bottom line. They consider how to lower expenses and raise revenue. Lowering expenses is very straightforward for these mega-farms: waste fewer crops every year. The less waste, the more they sell, the more money they make.

Fair enough. But *how* do they reduce waste? Now you're starting to ask the right questions! One of the major ways is the use of pesticides galore. Big Ag companies formulate chemical packages that are manufactured to kill insects, funguses, rodents, and weeds, and they spray them on and around the food that we end up eating. One of the most commonly used concoctions is called glyphosate (which is the primary herbicide in the common product Roundup). According to the Environmental Protection Agency (EPA), "about 280 million pounds of glyphosate are applied to an average of 298 million acres of cropland annually."[2] That's a whole lot of chemicals on a whole lot of crops. As Big Ag becomes more and more reliant on glyphosate, the weeds grow more and more resistant to the poison. The response? Genetic modifications to the crops (our food!) to strengthen their resistance to the glyphosate to allow Big Ag to spray more.

Can you spot the vicious cycle? The more they spray, the more they have to change the very makeup of our food, so they can spray more, to ultimately need to modify more. By the end of it, our food is unrecognizable. Consumers are eating pounds of chemicals off of mutated crops, and mega-farm corporations are getting richer.

Granted, the EPA goes through a review process and has stated, "Many pesticides can [indeed] pose risks to people. Generally, however, people are likely to be exposed to only very small amounts of pesticides—too small to pose a risk."[3] This would be reassuring, but the problem is that when products like pesticides are reviewed by the government for human health concerns, the government is looking only at immediate toxicity effects. They look at how the human body responds to interactions with the chemical directly, but they aren't considering the long-term effects of exposure to that chemical in almost everything we eat every day of our lives.

Eating these "conventionally" farmed foods won't immediately harm you in ways that you may expect if you swallowed a poison (what pesticides literally are). But chronic exposure to these chemicals has massive effects on the delicate balance of our microbiome. Consistent exposure to pesticides can lower bacteria diversity in the microbiome, raise microbiome toxicity, and affect the pathways that these bacteria take in metabolizing our food.[4] In short, what's killing those weeds is also killing our microbiomes. The trillions of bacteria living in us are sensitive, and, unfortunately, even a low dose of poison will wipe them out. This is to say nothing of studies that link chronic exposure to cancer and neurotoxicity.[5]

Essentially, our food has been poisoned.

If you don't believe any of that, believe this: Bayer (the maker of Roundup) has already announced they will no longer use glyphosate in residential herbicides because they have been sued over health damages so often.[6] However, there is no plan to stop using those 280 million pounds of glyphosate on our cropland. Out of sight, out of mind is their bet.

That's just one major (but not unique) example of dangerous cost-cutting across the Big Ag industry, but what about raising revenue? That brings us right back to the good ol' U.S. government. The government substantially subsidizes farms (with our tax dollars) in order to protect farms from disaster and keep food production steady during challenging economic times. Again, these are ideas that on their surface seem positive. I'm sure these subsidies started with the best of intentions. However, those intentions were also meant to be temporary. Those intentions were also meant for World War I. Seriously. These farm subsidies started to support ramped-up crop demand to support the Allies in the Great War. After the war ended, the expanded production didn't, because the money didn't either. Then the Great Depression hit, and more subsidies were used to maintain consistent yields. Then came World War II, and we were producing more than ever. Now these subsidies are so ingrained into our system that they simply can't be tamed.[7]

A two-pronged issue emerged: direct government aid accounts for 39% of net farm income (as of 2020)[8] and the government primarily subsidizes only a handful of "commodity" crops, such as wheat, corn, and soybeans. Mix those things together and you have a recipe for, well...wheat, corn, and soybeans. If you've ever driven through Kansas and wondered why there is so much corn, the answer is not for everyone's Fourth of July cookouts. Instead, it's because that's where all the money is. Have you ever asked yourself how we got to the point where the 1992 official food pyramid had a base of 6-11 servings of cereal-based products per day? Well, here is your answer: the echo chamber of subsidies, overproduction, and a need to sell it all to consumers. Essentially, we were told to build our diets around what they produced, not what would help us flourish.

Sadly, there aren't any significant subsidies for "specialty" crops (i.e. most fruits and vegetables), so farms don't grow them nearly as often. In fact, only 3% of farmland is used for them.[9] When farms choose to grow these crops, the produce ends up being much more expensive, because those farms don't have thirty-nine percent of their expenses paid for by the government. Instead, the cost is eaten (pun intended) by the consumer. Next time you complain that healthy food is so expensive, remember there are policies (that can be changed) causing that.

By the way, who is buying all that corn and soy anyway?!

You are. Because it's in *everything*.

High Fructose Corn Syrup. Soybean Oil. Corn Oil. Guar Gum. Natural Flavors. Citric Acid. Fructose. Corn Meal. Soy Lecithin. Cornstarch. Monosodium. Confectioner's Sugar. Maltodextrin.

These are just a *few* of the hiding places for that corn and soy in your ingredient labels.[10] These are mostly genetically modified, pesticide-covered, high-in-sugar, filler foods that continue to throw our guts out of balance. They aren't there for any nutrients they could offer but because they are cheap. This is particularly true for high fructose corn syrup and corn/soybean oil. High-quality, natural sugar and fat simply cost more than these cheap substitutes. From a business perspective, of course the cheaper option would win, as long as consumers keep buying it.

Even if you aren't eating those hidden soy and corn products, then maybe you're eating something that ate them. Soybeans and corn are two of the main ingredients in animal feed. When you eat the cow or chicken that ate this fake food, it's as though you were eating it yourself.

Why is this all happening? Because Big Ag had to figure out some way to use all the corn and soy they grew on the government's behalf. The government won't change the rules because the Big Ag's lobbyists have so much money from all the subsidies. It is a never-ending, broken cycle. And we, the consumers, are paying the highest cost of all: being stuck in a chronic imbalance leading to chronic inflammation and ultimately chronic disease that no one takes the blame for. If you're ever going to get out from under the broken system, it's going to be because you did something about it for yourself; Big Ag and food corporations won't do it for you. They're making too much money to care.

Part III

A Different Way

Part III
Introduction

Part II was not the most fun to research and write. No one wants to hear about all the ways we have damaged our relationship with food, which may be preventing us from flourishing in God's design. Maybe it was even more challenging to dip your toes into understanding the deceptive practices that mutate our food away from that good design. It can be shocking to learn that the food we grew up on (or maybe still eat) has been slowly killing us. Sometimes it feels like ignorance is bliss. But thankfully, it most certainly is not.

When it comes to rooting out any destructive practice in our lives, the first step is bringing it into the light. How can we change if we don't know the problem? Then, once we do know, we don't focus only on behavior modification. It is great to stop the negative action itself, but we'll only be able to grit it out for so long if we still long to jump back into it. Behavior modification hardly ever works long term. Heart modification does. Desire modification changes everything.

One humbling thing to remember is that this sort of heart change is only God's work. The Apostle Paul wrote:

> "For it is God who works in you, both to will and to work for His good pleasure."
>
> PHILIPPIANS 2:13

Don't attempt to do this in your own strength. Remember this is more than a physical exercise. It is a spiritual, emotional, and mental one, too. God wants to change your heart to yearn to live in His will and design.

Cry out to Him. Praise Him for the incredible gift of the food He has given us. Really examine yourself and consider if there have been potentially harmful motives behind your food choices. Even if not, ask Him to help you to flourish in His design. God loves to answer that prayer.

That is exactly why this book is structured the way it is. We started with the stunning beauty of God's incredible design for our bodies— how they are made to heal themselves and how God set up a system to do just that. We're not just learning to say "no" to things; we're saying "yes" to something far better.

Then, we turned our eyes to the pains of missed opportunities to flourish and the world's deceptive practices that make it more difficult to live in His design for our healing. If we don't know *why* we fall short, we'll never take the next step to flourish in His good design. Finally, we'll move into the practical "now what?" For any of this information to matter, there does need to be some real change. It can't simply stay in our heads; it must move to our hands.

These last chapters are not about a diet. Diets don't work because they are a battle we fight against what we really want. Diets live out of a scarcity mindset: "I can't have that" or "I really shouldn't." That is not what I would encourage. Instead, I hope to open our eyes to the abundance, beauty, and glory of living in God's design. I want you to live in freedom to celebrate both the food and healing that God wants us to enjoy. Haley and I absolutely love the rich, full, flavorful foods that we eat every day. It's not a burdensome obligation; it's a lifestyle we *choose* and *enjoy*. The more we walk in God's design for healing, the more we actually want to keep going.

The rest of this book will be the practical culmination of everything we've talked about thus far. What action steps do we take to mature in body and spirit? Spoiler alert: there are so many amazing ways! Some are simple, others are more difficult. Of course, this isn't intended to be a comprehensive list of all the possible ways to flourish. Rather, these final chapters provide concrete applications that you can actually try in your life. We'll start with food itself, then we'll discuss some practices that can be helpful. I don't expect each individual to fit every single suggestion into their lifestyle, but there are options throughout that would help anyone flourish. Some things will jive with certain people more. Have fun with trying new things! Don't try to do everything at once and overwhelm yourself. Take it day by day, step by step. Plant small habits and watch them grow into a flourishing lifestyle. The important thing is to move in the right direction. Let's take that first step together.

Chapter 12
The Foundations

In this chapter, we'll go through various quick-hit topics with some practical tips on how Haley and I have sought to live within God's healing design for each topic. The chapter is broken into smaller sections so that you can easily reference this information in the future. Use this as a guidebook to healing living. Of course, this is a very limited list and only a sampling of all the possibilities out there for living in God's flourishing design. Let it rev your creative engine to explore other topics that we don't discuss. But we need to start somewhere. You won't immediately do all of these perfectly. This is the culmination of years of seeking how to glorify God in our eating. And Haley and I are still learning more! But choose one topic and take a step in the right direction. These are some of the foundations that should help you build a lifestyle that continuously grows into His beautiful design.

Use Your Head

The first step is in some ways the easiest and in others the hardest: think before you eat. Don't just eat anything that is in front of you.

To be honest, this is still probably my biggest personal struggle with my relationship to food. I am far too easily pleased with free pizza or mac & cheese. If it's there, I'm probably eating it. Ironically, someone who's physical condition forces them to avoid certain foods has a bit of an advantage here. I certainly wouldn't choose a chronic disease but knowing that food would cause an immediate impact is a powerful deterrent. If you're like me and you don't have a diagnosed condition forcing you to avoid certain foods, then you're probably much more likely to fall prey to some of the traps we talked about in Part II.

The problem here is that every single one of us will feel the effects of the food we ingest. All of us. No exceptions. The only question is when it will happen. Will you feel that impact immediately, because your body has rejected low-quality food so many times that it has become chronically inflamed? Or will you feel it months, years, or decades down the road? It will catch up to you. Don't think that an "iron stomach" or "fast metabolism" will last forever. Don't be lulled into apathy because you haven't seen the consequences yet. That just guarantees nothing will change until you do.

A helpful tip if you struggle with saying "no" when junk food is in front of you is to make your home a safe place. Don't even allow foods that tempt you to enter that space. That way, when you're snacking or making dinner, your only options are healing ones. And when (not if) you do eat something that is hurtful rather than healing, don't beat yourself up. Remember, you're not trying to stay on a diet. You didn't break some arbitrary rule. Change the mindset to be more about wanting to help your body do its amazing healing work. If you ate something that hindered that, note it and move on.

Whole Foods (And I Don't Mean the Store)

When it comes to the question of what you should eat, the simplest answer is real, whole foods. What that means is, as much as possible, rather than eating processed foods that come out of a box or bag, eat foods that come straight from the ground, in their most natural form. Food helps our bodies thrive most when it is left untouched by machines, preservatives, and over-processing. That is how God designed it, so that's how we should enjoy it!

Another way of thinking about this is to eat *living* foods. Have you ever seen a potato chip sprout or a Chips Ahoy ripen? That's because the more you process the foods, the further from their living self they become. When they lose that life, they lose their nutrients, too. Living foods are teaming with cells, vitamins, minerals, and even good bacteria that are healing for our bodies. They maintain life for the plant or animal, and now they can help maintain that life for us! Living foods help you live. Dead foods help you die. It really is that simple.

Typically, you'll find these living, whole foods on the perimeter of the grocery store. That's because living food doesn't last long enough to store it in those non-refrigerated middle aisles. Instead, those aisles are the packaged and processed food realm. Try to limit what you get from that middle area. Of course, the farmer's market is going to sell almost entirely whole, living foods. Look for things like fresh produce, meats, herbs, nuts, seeds, and mushrooms. We'll look more into some specifics throughout the chapter.

Go Organic

As simple as it sounds, veggies, fruits, and meats are really the pillars for a flourishing body. But not all produce and meats are created equal. Part II went into detail about the nasty stuff that goes on at Big Ag farms. Unfortunately, the reality is that those corporate farms produce a majority of the food we buy from grocery stores. That is why it is so vital to eat organic. I've heard the old arguments like "Organic is just a scam to get you to pay more money for the same stuff", or "You can't even taste the difference between organic and regular produce." I get it. I used to have those same thoughts myself. I was shocked when I learned that organic food isn't actually supposed to taste different. Who knew?! However, even though the taste is similar, that doesn't mean it isn't wildly different from so-called conventional foods.

The truth is certified organic produce (according to the USDA) is "grown on soil that had no prohibited substances applied for three years prior to harvest. Prohibited substances include most synthetic fertilizers and pesticides."[1] This includes the dangerous pesticide mentioned in Chapter 11, glyphosate. The USDA's definition also prohibits certain agricultural practices. One important prohibited practice is the use of any genetically modified organisms. Certified organic ingredients also can't be treated with radiation or sewage sludge. You would think that would be common sense applied to all of our food suppliers, but it must've been common enough to need to be included in the rules.

Crazy.

Perhaps the government can't be fully trusted to treat food the way that it was designed to be treated. The USDA organic system isn't flawless. But it is undoubtedly a major step up from conventional produce, which is likely covered in synthetic chemicals, genetically modified, and even exposed to sewage sludge. The less your food is impacted by those things, the less your gut and microbiome have to deal with the aftermath.

A non-profit called the Environmental Working Group puts out an annual list of the foods that are most sprayed with pesticides called the "Dirty Dozen."[2] That's a great place to start when deciding which items you'll begin to switch out first. These top offenders are usually berries, leafy greens, bell peppers, and other foods without a protective husk (as opposed to fruits like watermelon and pineapple which have that outer layer). At least commit to switching out those top offenders for organic versions. You may not feel an immediate impact of the change, but you will be laying the foundation for your body to rest, heal, and fight disease.

Organic + Local Is the Perfect Pair

I want to clarify that eating local and eating organic are not the same thing. There are local farms that use plenty of pesticides. There are farms on the other side of the world that are organic. Personally, I believe prioritizing organic practices is the most important piece because of the intense damage that consistent pesticide ingestion can cause. That said, the ideal practice would be to source organically grown produce from a local farm. The great news is that many local farms are doing it right, even if they aren't certified organic (many farms use organic practices but don't pay for the certification).

The advantages of sourcing locally are many. For one, you get your food from someone you know and trust. You have a real person you can talk to and ask them about their practices. You can ask what foods are grown at what time of the year, why, and how. Here's a wild idea: you could actually visit the place your food is grown! Farmers that own and run small farms likely care a lot more about the well-being of their crops and livestock than an industrially run option, so their product is often higher quality. The smaller scale of local farms lessens dependency on harmful practices and increases the farmer's ability to lend an intentional eye. The economics matter, too. Every dollar you give to a small-scale, local, organic farm is a dollar that doesn't go to the Big Ag machine. Spending local supports local, and in a world that leans towards corporate consolidation, every dollar counts. Finally, and perhaps most importantly, nutrient availability in foods often begins decreasing as soon as the food is harvested.[3] Therefore, the less the time from harvest to your plate, the more nutrients your food will maintain.

Veggies

When it comes to vegetables, I've heard many people claim not to like the taste of them. I truly believe this is not because God's food tastes bad, but because our pervasive desires for convenience and cutting costs have done damage. What I mean is that in an attempt to keep things cheap and fast, our veggies have been canned, boiled, and microwaved. Repeated horrible experiences with mushy, overcooked veggies have left a literal bad taste in our mouths. Here we have yet another reason to eat whole foods rather than the bagged or canned versions: they taste a million times better.

I've found that just about any veggie—green beans, asparagus, brussels sprouts, butternut squash, beets, etc.—taste amazing with a drizzle of olive oil, salt, pepper, garlic powder and are roasted in the oven on 385°F for 15-20 minutes (add some time for denser veggies like beets). I mean, seriously, they have so much natural flavor, and any bitterness is roasted out into crispy goodness.

Sautéing is another quick way to lock in flavor and prevent unappetizing mushiness. The key, whether roasting or sautéing, is cooking with a high-quality fat (more on these in a moment). As you cook with higher temperatures, you'll want to use saturated fats like grass-fed butter or coconut oil, which are more stable at high heat. These high-quality fats also taste wonderful and have their own benefits for your body.

Cooking the veggies is also particularly helpful if you have concerns about your gut, as it helps begin to break down the food before you eat it. Often raw veggies can be harder on the digestive system, especially if your system is already struggling. Making veggies that you actually enjoy is simpler than you may think. You don't need complicated recipes or special equipment. You just need high-quality produce, fat, and heat.

Green juices are another amazing and practical way of getting your vegetables in. They are particularly helpful because your body doesn't need to digest any solids, so your body can absorb the nutrients much quicker. Just be sure to get green juices that are low in sugar (many add pineapple or apple juice, which have a lot of sugar), cold-pressed/unpasteurized (to make sure the nutrients stay intact), and organic (so you aren't absorbing chemical toxins along with your juice). Drinking a green juice in the morning before eating can allow the nutrients to be absorbed quickly and potently. These juices are more of an acquired taste, but with some consistency you'll come to love them!

Fruits

Of course, you can't have vegetables without their sister—fruit! God's natural dessert and sweeteners are also packed with incredible nutrients. Even though fruits are higher in sugar content, over-indulging in their natural, unrefined sugar is much more difficult to do than with the processed sugars we typically eat. That's because the natural fiber in fruit fills you up before you eat too much. Shift your fruit with the seasons. For example, enjoy the incredible antioxidants of berry season in the summer and the immune-boosting citruses of winter. Avoid buying fruits out of season as they need to be shipped across the world to get to your grocery store. These fruits were likely artificially ripened off the stem, and the long trip can be detrimental for them. A better option is to freeze in-season fruit so you can enjoy it all year long.

Smoothies are such an efficient and powerful way to get nutrients. They use the entire fruit, which means you get the fiber you miss out on in fruit juices. Mix and match fruits and find things you get excited to gulp down. Once you've decided on the fruit, add in a liquid base (like coconut water or raw milk—more on this in the next chapter), a handful or two of leafy greens (such as kale or spinach), maybe a nut butter (where the *only* ingredient is the nut), and even some natural sweetener (like honey or dates). No recipe here, just have fun! If you don't like it, keep blending until you do.

Just be careful that you're not adding ingredients with lots of added refined sugar, preservatives, or emulsifying additives. Particular products to check the ingredient labels for additives include alternative milks, fruit juices (avoid from concentrate), and flavored yogurts. For example, Almond Breeze's almond milk includes ingredients like potassium citrate and gellan gum.[4] Some alternative milks (especially oat) even contain canola oil—a genetically-modified, chemically-extracted, seed-based oil. Most store-bought flavored yogurts are loaded with added refined sugar, even seemingly simple flavors like vanilla. Don't counteract the natural goodness of your smoothie with chemicals or unnecessary added sugar!

Then, the secret ingredient for an amazing, healing smoothie is a superfood or two. These are nutrient-dense foods that you wouldn't ordinarily eat but really support your body's flourishing. Typically, you find them in dried and powdered form. It could be reishi mushroom, spirulina, açaí, ashwagandha, goji berries, chia seeds, collagen, and more. There are tons of options that take your smoothie to the next level.

Support The Microbiome

Part of the reason organic fruits and veggies are so important is that many of them contain what is called *pre*biotics. These prebiotics are primarily dietary fiber, which is typically present in fruits and veggies. Essentially, prebiotics are not only food for us but also food for the good bacteria in our gut that make up our microbiome. The more prebiotics you eat, the more fuel you give your microbiome and, consequently, the more effectively your digestive and immune systems work. If you aren't getting a healthy amount of these prebiotics in your diet, then inflammation can begin to take root and lead to chronic disease.

Once your diet has sufficient prebiotics, you'll also want to think about how to incorporate lots of good *pro*biotics as well! When you hear that word, you may automatically think about a pill. While supplements can be helpful (we'll talk more about these later), they are not the only (or even the best) way to get probiotics. Lots of foods are naturally probiotic, meaning they have good, living bacteria in them which help heal and maintain gut health. A key place to look for probiotics is in fermented foods (think kombucha—fermented tea; sauerkraut—fermented cabbage; and yogurt—fermented milk). These are great examples of how bacteria can be our friend. The bacteria in these foods both preserve it naturally and they directly support our gut—and therefore our immune and digestive systems. Fermented foods aren't the most popular in Western culture, but they are some of the healthiest options you can eat.

Meat

When it comes to meat, quality is the number one factor to consider. No matter what kind of animal our meats are sourced from, they are better for us if they live a healthy life themselves. This means that you want meat from animals that lived as close to their natural, wild life as possible. Otherwise, you'll simply be consuming the by-product of their pesticide-covered corn and soy feed, which isn't good for anyone.

For red meat, look for grass-fed *and* finished cows. If they don't *finish* the cow with grass, then at the end of their life, the cows are fattened up with the same animal feed that we are looking to avoid. One study reviewed three decades of research and concluded that on a gram-for-gram basis, compared to grain-fed beef, grass-fed beef has:

- A more ideal omega-3 to omega-6 ratio
- More vitamin A
- More vitamin E
- More cancer-fighting antioxidants like glutathione
- Lower total fat content[5]

There is an undeniable link between our food's health and ours! In fact, you could argue that grass-fed beef is biblical. I submit to you Psalm 104:14:

> "You cause *grass* to grow for the livestock and plants for people to use. You allow them to produce food from the earth."

God caused grass to grow for the cows, not corn or soy! Corn and soy-fed beef contains a concerningly high ratio of omega-6 to omega-3 that can lead to inflammation in the gut. On the other hand, grass-fed beef's much higher omega-3 and antioxidant content can actually give it an *anti*-inflammatory effect. This isn't a trivial difference.

For chicken, look for pasture-raised chicken. Be careful not to be fooled by "free range" chicken, which just requires outdoor access, whereas pasture-raised means they actually live outdoors on at least 2.5 acres of land.[6] Try venturing out from just boneless, skinless chicken breasts. Consider buying a whole chicken from the farmers market and roast it. Eat some of the dark meat and the skin. Save the bones to make homemade bone broth, something that is especially easy to do with an Instant Pot.

Bone broth is made by simmering chicken bones so long that the natural vitamins, minerals, and collagen within it become highly concentrated in the broth. In fact, since it's both full of protein and is naturally anti-inflammatory, a bone broth fast may even be a possible healing route if you are in a place of major digestive issues. Haley and I try to keep bone broth (either in soup or simply drinking it) as a consistent part of our diet.

Pork can either be labeled as grass-fed or pasture-raised, both of which are good indicators. Uncured pork bacon (yes, bacon!) or sausage from our local farm are some of our go-to breakfast meats. Chorizo is an absolute favorite. Just make sure to read the ingredients to check for any chemical, preservative, or sugar additives. All the ingredients listed should be foods that you would eat by themselves!

When it comes to fish, look for "wild caught"—which means exactly what it sounds like. Farm-raised fish (the opposite of wild caught) are fed diets which can include corn/soy products and may even have added dyes to give them the hue they would have in the wild. Salmon (and other fish) help us flourish because they are high in omega-3 fatty acids, which the National Institutes of Health note "are important components of the membranes that surround each cell in your body." They go on to say that omega-3 fatty acids support "functions in your heart, blood vessels, lungs, immune system, and endocrine system (the network of hormone-producing glands)."[7] If possible, shoot for Alaskan-caught fish as Atlantic-caught fish may have higher rates of chemical exposure.

Lastly, it's worth mentioning that muscle meat (the vast majority of meat in the American diet) is not the only type of meat. In fact, organ meat is perhaps one of the most nutritious foods we can eat. Nutrients that many Americans are deficient in like vitamin A, a variety of B vitamins, iron, copper, and choline are prevalent in organ meats like liver. A recent study sought to identify which foods would best fill a typical adult's nutrient gaps in the least number of calories. The answer? Four out of the top seven best options were organ meats (specifically liver, spleen, kidney, and heart, in that order).[8] I realize that may not be enough to get you to try it, but those results are quite compelling.

Chicken liver is probably the easiest entry point into organ meat, but beef liver is also highly nutritious. You can start by mixing it into any dish which uses ground beef or simply pan-fry it and eat it on its own. Pro tip: soak the liver in milk before cooking to make it significantly more palatable. Another option is cutting it into small pieces, freezing it, and swallowing it like a pill if you really can't stand the taste. Our ancestors never wasted any piece of the animal and were better off for it. Organ meats are one way we can emulate that in our lives.

Of course, wherever you can, buy your meat organic, which the USDA defines as "animals [that] are raised in living conditions accommodating their natural behaviors (like the ability to graze on pasture), fed 100% organic feed and forage, and not administered antibiotics or hormones."[9] Finding a local farm which holds to these standards for your meat is ideal. The treatment of the animal in their lifetime is so vital and it's something that may only truly be possible on a small-scale farm. Even the best-intended industrial meat farms are simply not able to maintain the level of intentional care needed for this quality of meat. The further you get from the industrial meat industry the better. On the flip side, the closer you get to your local farmer the better.

High-quality meats are not only okay to eat, but they are actually helpful to your overall health. Not to mention, they taste a whole lot better than industrial meats or meat substitutes. God has allowed us to eat meat ever since we left the Garden of Eden, after all!

High-Quality Fats

Just as animal proteins have their place, so do animal fats. Animal fats often have nutrients that are hard to find in other places. For example, butter has a high amount of vitamin A and E plus a compound called butyrate, which has been linked to microbiome support and reduced inflammation.[10] Grass-fed tallow (rendered beef fat) is also high in many nutrients that are hard to find like Vitamin A and D. Simply put, without enjoying some of these animal-based foods (meats, organs, and fats), there are essential nutrients in which we will almost certainly be deficient.

There are also wonderful plant-based fats like olive, coconut, and avocado oils that help your body flourish. What makes olive, coconut, and avocado oils different from other plant-based oils is that they are squeezed from the fatty *fruit* of the plant. A good quality form of these oils has only minimal processing because extracting the oil only takes a simple pressing technique. On the contrary, industrial seed-based or so-called vegetable oils take massive refining efforts to reach a point where they can be used.

Thankfully, recent studies have started to debunk the "saturated fats (mostly animal fats) are bad" and "unsaturated fats (mostly vegetable oils) are good" narrative. One study's conclusion went as far as to conclude, "Current evidence does not clearly support cardio-vascular guidelines that encourage high consumption of poly-unsaturated fatty acids and low consumption of total saturated fats."[11]

Any given fat is made up of some combination of saturated fat, monounsaturated fat, or polyunsaturated fat which "differ by the number of double bonds their chemical structures contain."[12] Basically, these double bonds are prone to deterioration by interaction with oxygen, a process called oxidation. In fact, this is exactly why you've probably heard that antioxidants are great for your health; they are anti-oxidation. Polyunsaturated fats ("poly" meaning more than one double bond) are the most at risk of oxidation, given the greater number of double bonds they have. Then, when your body uses this fat to build your cells, those cells are more at risk of deterioration, too.

There are two types of polyunsaturated fats, omega-6s and omega-3s. The ratio of omega-6s to omega-3s is another consideration in choosing the right fats. Since mankind started squeezing oils from seeds, we've consumed far more omega-6s than the rest of human history. It's estimated that our omega-6 to omega-3 ratio has gone from around 1:1 to about 20:1 in the last hundred years.[13] While omega-6 is an important nutrient, this level of change cannot be healthy. Again, industrial oils like canola, cottonseed, soybean, corn, and sunflower are particularly high in omega-6s, while coconut oil, olive oil, butter, tallow, and other animal fats are typically lower in omega-6s. We need the right balance of saturated, mono-unsaturated, and polyunsaturated fats in our lives, and we need them from quality sources. Practically, this means limiting poly-unsaturated fats from highly processed seed and vegetable oils and increasing high-quality animal fats.

For animal fats, follow the same guidelines as you would for other animal products. Look for fats from grass-fed or pasture-raised animals. You can even render your own version of tallow by saving the drippings of cooked ground beef and letting it solidify (a great way to save money). Don't be afraid of animal-based, saturated fats. Contrary to what we've been told, they can actually be beneficial for our bodies and are certainly a better alternative to industrial seed oils.

For plant-based fats, stay away from anything hydrogenated, which often contains trans fat. Rather than cooking with canola, sunflower, or just general vegetable oil, replace those with olive, avocado, or coconut oil. Look for the "raw" or "extra virgin" label to ensure minimal processing. Get both animal and plant fats organic and from as close to home as possible.

While what you use at home to cook with is important, most of these low-quality oils show up in processed food or even most restaurant food. Unless a restaurant explicitly tells you that they are *not* using industrial seed-based oils, it is safe to assume they *are* using them. Even if they tell you they are using something like olive oil, that may be a blend of olive oil and an industrial seed-based oil. Unfortunately, many seemingly "healthy" options at restaurants (think: salad dressing or grilled chicken) are covered in these poor quality oils. Industrial oils are simply too cheap for most businesses to pass up. This is another reason that cooking most meals at home is so important to overall health.

High-quality fat can support brain, immune, and gut health; over-processed industrial fat can destroy those. Make an effort to know the quality of the fats you're consuming so that they work for you and not against you.

Water

To close out our foundations chapter, we'll look at perhaps the most obvious building block of all: water. Our bodies are mostly water, so filling them with good, clean water is essential. Don't settle for municipal water from the tap. Your city's water treatment plant does not do enough for your water. There are tons of dissolved solids lurking in your tap water. There is often leftover residue of prescription drugs and other nasty things that contaminate our water system. For example, my zip code's tap water contains high levels of bromodichloromethane, chloroform, and haloacetic acids.[14] You can check your zip code's tap water at *www.ewg.org/tapwater*. Use a water filter that targets these contaminants, not just improves taste.

We have come to love the Zero Filter (no sponsorship here!), which removes all dissolved solids including lead, arsenic, mercury, and asbestos. It also comes with a meter that lets you test your water for dissolved solids. Then you can really see the difference the filter is making.

Drink water early and often. Start your day off with a big glass of water to get the wheels of your body moving. Keep a reusable (preferably not plastic) water bottle full and near you so you can drink when you're bored. The rule of thumb is to drink half your body weight in ounces, though that's not something I personally track. Consistency is more important than hitting a target. Drinking lots of water keeps your body flowing, preventing stagnation in your gut. Adding a pinch of pink sea salt or a squeeze of lemon juice adds some natural electrolytes, particularly useful after a big sweat. Other drinks that are naturally high in electrolytes (and therefore highly hydrating) include coconut water and raw milk.

Closing Thoughts

I can understand if all of that is a bit overwhelming. I don't intend to bombard you. Remember that this chapter is also designed as a reference guide for when you have questions on individual topics in the future. Rather than implementing every one of those recommendations, what I hope is that you are able to take just one step towards changing your relationship with food. Out of all the topics you have just read about, pick the one that got you the most excited and focus on that to start. I truly believe that as you see your body flourish in God's good design, you will *want* to try the next one. Then it's no longer a burden but a joy.

If you have to start somewhere, maybe consider what you're eating a little bit more each time you order out or go to the grocery store. Or you could think a little more about how the food got from where it started to your plate. The way your food is made is almost as important as what kind of food it is. Seek to grow in your understanding of what is truly nourishing. It can be as simple as just listening to your body. Or getting to know a farmer. Or buying local. Or going organic. In summation, eat what God gave us.

Chapter 13
The Threats

Last chapter mostly focused on some great things we can *add* to our dietary habits, but we all have things we need to limit, too. That's what this chapter is about: the threats to our healing potential. Remember, I'm not giving you a prescription for what to eat and what not to eat. If you eat something that you know you shouldn't, you're not "cheating." It doesn't mean you've failed or that you have to start from square one. My hope is that you understand *why* you should want to eat certain things and *why* you should want to avoid certain things. That is *so much* more powerful than a list of forbidden foods.

The more your eyes are opened, the more your desires will change. The more you see God's design for food, the more you'll look at a bag of Skittles and think to yourself, "I genuinely don't want to put my body through that." Start enjoying the real food from the last chapter and start to witness these changes in your desires. It won't happen immediately; it's a process and a journey, so keep taking it one step at a time. I think that is the way God meant it to be. That's how He designed growth to work in our spiritual lives in general. We don't have all the answers and we certainly make mistakes, but He cares more about us taking the next step to know Him deeper than He does about us checking the boxes. If you are genuinely looking to grow, in faith or in healing, I think you're headed in the right direction.

Ultra-Processed Foods

As the antithesis to one of the main ideas of the last chapter (eat real, whole foods), the logical first recommendation for threats to avoid is ultra-processed foods. Now, the technical definition of processed foods would include food that's been through *any* sort of process, even something like pre-washing vegetables. There are ancient processes that can actually increase the healing potential of our foods, like the fermentation we discussed last chapter. Basically, when I say ultra-processed foods, I mean the "multi-ingredient industrially formulated mixes" we examined in Part II. These are typically foods you buy in boxes or bags that come ready to eat and never go bad. But not every boxed or bagged option is created equal. So, for the cases where you feel an ultra-processed food is necessary, let's consider how to choose the best options for you and your family.

Read The Ingredients

One of the most practical steps to take is to simply read the label. And I don't mean the calorie content. In fact, I rarely look at the Nutrition Facts. Instead, focus on the ingredients. If what you're eating is made up of real food, then the number of calories or carbs doesn't matter nearly as much. Don't fall for marketing schemes and colorful logos. Care about the actual contents. For example, even just a glance at the ingredients in Skittles should raise major red flags as you'd see: sugar, corn syrup, hydrogenated palm kernel oil, modified corn starch, natural flavors, artificial flavors, and a bunch of synthetic food dyes.[1] Let's take a deeper look at those ingredients.

First of all, sugar is the main ingredient, but let's even move past that (I mean, it is a candy after all). Next, you see corn syrup and modified corn starch later down the list. If you read Part II of this book, then your spidey-sense should be tingling. These are ingredients Big Ag mass produces because of the enormous incentives they have to produce corn, which is positively covered in pesticides and chemicals before being processed to the point of not even being recognizable as a plant. Next, you see the hydrogenated palm kernel oil, which was developed as a poor attempt to replace synthetic trans fat (only when the FDA forced this change on food producers). Two key words here are *hydrogenated* and *kernel*. Hydrogenated is a major red flag. We briefly discussed in Part II how hydrogenation is a process that changes vegetable oils to act like animal fats. This transformation of the fat means there are some levels of trans fat in these products, even if they don't show up on the label. The other keyword, *kernel*, means it's from the seed, not the fruit of the plant. This essentially guarantees serious processing (think: harsh chemical solvents) was necessary to extract the oil.

Then you take a look at the synthetic additives: natural flavors, artificial flavors, and food dyes. We learned earlier that the "natural" versions of these flavors are likely also hidden corn products with the same issues mentioned before. The artificial version doesn't even try to hide the fact that it ain't food. The FDA defines artificial flavors as "any substance, the function of which is to impart flavor, which is *not* derived from a spice, fruit or fruit juice, vegetable or vegetable juice, edible yeast, herb, bark, bud, root, leaf or similar plant material, meat, fish, poultry, eggs, dairy products, or fermentation products thereof."[2] I mean, what else is there?! It is purely a chemical additive that your body was not designed to digest.

With a little bit of knowledge, care, and effort, you just went from downing a bag of Skittles without thinking to maybe a bit of a changed desire. Perhaps you don't actually want that bag of artificial inflammation bombs. That's the key. Learn, care, and try.

Find A Better Alternative

Now, I realize that the previous example was a bag of candy. I get it, we all know candy doesn't help our bodies flourish. But there are tons of other highly processed foods that we should avoid. The classic, and I think very effective, rule of thumb is to not eat anything you can't pronounce. This may not always be perfect, but it is a great starting place.

The next step is to identify some of the industry tricks (like natural and artificial flavors, vegetable oil, etc.) and avoid them. Thirdly, decide where it is absolutely necessary to include some highly processed (boxed or bagged) food in your diet and find one that you can feel good about. Ultra-processed foods shouldn't be the baseline, but the exception. Wherever you make the exception, choose a high-quality option. There are certainly better and worse options out there. As with anything, practice makes perfect. The more you understand the labeling, the quicker you'll be able to identify products you can eat with a clear conscience. For example, compare the ingredients of Wheat Thins and Simple Mills Crackers:

Wheat Thins[3]	Simple Mills Crackers[4]
Base	
Whole Grain Wheat Flour	Nut and Seed Flour Blend (Almonds, Sunflower, Flax Seeds)
	Cassava Flour
Fat	
Canola Oil	Organic Sunflower Oil
Flavoring	
Sugar	Organic Onion
Malt Syrup (From Corn and Barley)	Organic Garlic
Refiner's Syrup	Sea Salt
Salt	
Leavening/Thickening	
Cornstarch	Tapioca
Leavening (Calcium Phosphate and Baking Soda)	
Preservatives	
BHT Added to Packaging Material to Preserve Freshness	Rosemary Extract (For Freshness)

Comparing these two lists of ingredients, you can begin to notice a few major differences. The first category is the base of each cracker.

Wheat Thins	Simple Mills Crackers
Base	
Whole Grain Wheat Flour	Nut and Seed Flour Blend (Almonds, Sunflower, Flax Seeds)
	Cassava Flour

To Wheat Thins' credit, they do use whole grain wheat flour. We'll talk more about grains in a minute, but this isn't a horrible option. Of course, they market this one ingredient like crazy because it gives the appearance of a healthy snack. What's also important to remember is that wheat is one of the so-called commodity crops that the government subsidizes. This basically means that most of our wheat comes from massive farms using huge amounts of pesticides. So, this is a particular instance where not being organic has serious repercussions.

Simple Mills uses a nut, seed, and cassava mix. Almonds, sunflower seeds, and flax seeds each have their own nutrient profiles. For example, almonds are high in protein, vitamin E, and manganese, while flax seeds provide omega-3 fatty acids. Cassava flour comes from the cassava root, which is a popular gluten-free flour option. Of course, I would prefer these to be organic, so Simple Mills isn't perfect either. However, given the choice between non-organic wheat and non-organic nut and seed flour, the nut/seed is likely the better option.

Wheat Thins	Simple Mills Crackers
Fat	
Canola Oil	Organic Sunflower Oil

The oils are a big differentiator here. As mentioned in the last chapter, these types of oils are commonplace in packaged food. Both of our examples use a seed-based oil, but that doesn't make them equal. Canola oil is an absolute mess of genetically modified seeds from the rapeseed (yeah, bad name) plant. It is the poster child of these recently invented seed oils, having been created as late as 1974. Fun fact: the "can" in canola is short for Canada, where it was invented. It's a failed science experiment that does not qualify as nutritious, even though it's in most of our food. The Simple Mills crackers aren't perfect either. I'd prefer one of the higher quality fats we talked about in the last chapter. Sunflower oil is still a seed-based oil that requires chemical processing to extract and can be too high in omega-6 fatty acids. Although, there is significant comfort in knowing that this particular sunflower oil is organic, because that guarantees no genetic modifications or chemical pesticides.

Wheat Thins	Simple Mills Crackers
Flavoring	
Sugar	Organic Onion
Malt Syrup (From Corn and Barley)	Organic Garlic
Refiner's Syrup	Sea Salt
Salt	

Next, how is it that these two crackers are being flavored? For Simple Mills, that answer is fairly straightforward: they are flavored with organic onion and garlic with a touch of sea salt. For the Wheat Thins, it's a little less clear where the flavor is coming from, but the answer is truly *sugar*.

Sugar itself is one of the ingredients. Also included is "Malt Syrup (From Corn and Barley)", which would perhaps be okay if it were made only with high-quality barley, but you'll notice the label says it's—once again—made with corn. That means it's essentially corn syrup. By now you know what corn syrup is—more sugar. With that, "Refiner's Syrup" is just another form of sugar (it even tells you it's refined). Even in a product that most people wouldn't consider "sweet", sugar is lurking everywhere.

Next, we'll dive into the Leavening/Thickening and Preservatives categories, two areas where ingredients are often hard to decipher.

Wheat Thins	Simple Mills Crackers
Leavening/Thickening	
Cornstarch	Tapioca
Leavening (Calcium Phosphate and Baking Soda)	

As for leavening and thickening products, you see our good (or should I say bad?) friend, corn, shows up again in the Wheat Thins' cornstarch. They continue to find new creative ways to use that cheap corn! While calcium and phosphorus are both naturally occurring elements, when listed as an ingredient on their own, they are likely inorganic versions of these elements. Tapioca, on the other hand, is made from the cassava plant. Though it does go through a few processing steps to be used as a thickening agent, it is a far better alternative to the Wheat Thin options.

Wheat Thins	Simple Mills Crackers
Preservatives	
BHT Added to Packaging Material to Preserve Freshness	Rosemary Extract (For Freshness)

Lastly, let's check out the preservatives. Since both of these products use unsaturated fats, both companies needed to find a way to help prevent the oxidation that will turn that oil into a dangerous, rancid mess. For Wheat Thins, they chose to use BHT in the packaging. BHT, or butylated hydroxytoluene, is a synthetic preservative closely related to butylated hydroxyanisole which is "reasonably anticipated to be a human carcinogen" according to our very own U.S. government.[5] Not what you want in your food. Simple Mills had to solve a similar preservation problem, but they used a natural ingredient, rosemary extract. Rosemary has strong antioxidant properties, effectively preserving the crackers. It's likely that rosemary was more expensive than Wheat Thins' butylated hydroxytoluene, but it also doesn't cause cancer.

Priorities.

My hope in doing that exercise is to start to develop your skill of reading the language of the ingredient lists. Knowledge is power and there is so much hidden in the labels of processed foods. In a perfect world, we would avoid ultra-processed foods altogether, but when you do choose a highly processed option, be mindful about what ingredients are making up that product. Make an informed choice about what you're putting into your body. Find treats that you can both enjoy and feel good about eating.

Other Heavy Hitters

After processed foods, there are three other categories of foods that are smart to be extra mindful about. I do believe there are natural forms of each of these that are perfectly fine (or even helpful) to include in your lifestyle. However, the run-of-the-mill versions of these foods are tough to digest, and they tend to promote imbalance in our guts.

Those foods are sugar, grains, and dairy. These probably aren't a huge surprise. Sugar is demonized no matter who you ask. Of course, we've been seeing more and more gluten-free and dairy-free people these days—often by necessity instead of choice. That shouldn't shock us. Sugar, grains, and dairy are some of the most mutilated foods in our Western diet. Truly, the reason each of these is inflammatory and destroys our gut is because they're actually just a subset of our first category, ultra-processed foods.

Sugar

Let's start with sugar. We've already talked a bit about this one (especially some of the ultra-processed forms like high fructose corn syrup), but basically, we've been trained to be addicted to the stuff. The processed sugar that is far too normal these days does nothing positive for our body, but instead it can destroy our microbiome.

As much as you possibly can, avoid refined sugars and replace them with natural versions. Essentially, refined means that the naturally occurring sugars in a plant were ripped out and processed to be added into other foods and drinks. If God didn't put the sugar in there, it is likely refined.

Don't replace refined sugars with artificial sweeteners (such as aspartame) that present their own laundry list of problems. Rather than list out potential side effects, I'll point you back to the idea that God designed our food, including the sweet parts, perfectly. Replacing it with chemicals from a lab isn't the way to live out His design.

As best as you can, completely remove products that contain high fructose corn syrup. There is essentially no nutritional value in this sweet goo that is gathered from pesticide-covered crops. It's about as bad as it gets. For example, the "sports drink" Powerade is essentially water and high fructose corn syrup with 34 grams of sugar in a 28-ounce bottle.[6] A 20-ounce Coke is also essentially just water and corn syrup, in this case with a whopping 65 grams of sugar.[7] Cutting out high fructose corn syrup is an excellent place to start your healing journey, partly because of how prevalent it is in our food supply. You'll automatically be cutting out many processed foods and tons of refined sugar.

The easiest way to identify a product with refined sugar is to look at the "Added Sugar" line on the nutrition label. Generally, if it isn't added sugar, then it's naturally occurring in the ingredients, rather than refined.

As often as possible, get your sugar fix from whole fruits. The natural ratio of sugar to fiber helps your body assimilate the unrefined sweetness much better than its refined counterpart. Those same fibers also give the sensation of being full, so you'll be less likely to overeat whole fruit. You'll also be gaining the beneficial vitamins, antioxidants, and other properties fruit has to offer.

Besides fruit, look into dates, raw honey, pure maple syrup, and coconut sugar as alternatives. Raw honey has wonderful antifungal properties and if it's bought locally can help with seasonal allergies. Real maple syrup has antioxidants and vitamins that at least give it some nutritional value aside from the sweetness. Don't be fooled into thinking that most pancake syrups are real maple syrup. In fact, most of them don't even claim to be "maple" syrup, instead just "syrup." I'll give you three guesses at what kind of "syrup" they are made of. Hint: it starts with "high" and comes from corn.

As you begin to enjoy sweet foods in this new way, let your body adjust to a lower intake of sugar. Let your taste buds be okay with desserts that have more than one dimension (i.e. overwhelmingly sweet). It will take time and effort because of the unfathomable pervasion that sugar has in our diets. That's okay. Give it time. This one change can have a massive effect on your health and, depending on your current diet, you may feel very immediate impacts. Remember, God was the one who designed sweetness to be enjoyed in its time and place. You aren't missing out by enjoying it in His design. In fact, you'll likely realize that you've been missing out by indulging in the fake sweetness of the world.

Grains

So many people are moving towards a gluten-free lifestyle because they can feel their bodies rejecting the processed grains that make up most gluten-filled items like bread, baked goods, pasta, or beer. Once humans found a way to process grains quickly, cheaply, and with shelf-life, these processed grains became a staple in American homes, but their devastation on our health is hard to miss. The Harvard School for Public Health puts it like this:

> "The invention of industrialized roller mills in the late 19th century changed the way we process grains. Milling strips away the bran and germ and leaves only the soft, easy-to-digest endosperm. Without the fibrous bran, the grain is easier to chew. The germ is removed because of its fat content, which can limit the shelf life of processed wheat products. The resulting highly processed grains are much lower in nutritional quality. Refining wheat creates fluffy flour that makes light, airy breads and pastries, but the process strips away more than half of wheat's B vitamins, 90 percent of the vitamin E, and virtually all of the fiber."[8]

If you've ever wondered why so many boxed and bagged grain-based products use "enriched" flour, it's not because they want you to get your vitamins. It's because they've mangled the flour so much it has nothing left in it. Grains are not inherently bad for you, not at all. However, nearly all grain-based foods you can find these days are so processed they are destroying your gut health.

For this reason, limiting grains in your diet may be helpful. However, if you do eat grains, go for organic, sprouted, whole-grain versions. Organic is particularly important for wheat products as it is one of those commodity crops that gets drenched in pesticides. Sprouted means they soak the grain seed until it just begins to grow. That means it's still alive! And to be alive it needs to be whole (meaning it has all three parts still: bran, germ, and endosperm). Since the grain is alive, it starts to release enzymes and nutrients to support itself, which means those nutrients are available for our bodies in a way you just can't get in dead grains.[9] In fact, these enzymes even start to break down the gluten, so people with intolerances may have a better experience with sprouted whole grain! A true long-fermented sourdough made with organic ingredients (preferably homemade) is about as good as you can get when it comes to bread. The long-fermentation process significantly improves the digestibility of the gluten.

Oats can be one of the most nutritious grains we can eat, but please don't think that instant microwave oatmeal is providing you anything in the way of healing. The least processed version of oats is the steel-cut version. A great breakfast option is overnight prepared steel-cut oats. Letting them soak overnight helps with digestion and makes cooking them much quicker. Like wheat, oats are also notorious for being heavily sprayed with pesticides, so put them on the urgent list for buying organic. Big Ag farms will actually spray a heavy dose of glyphosate on both wheat and oats directly before harvesting to intentionally kill the crops. The point is that the dead crops dry out and are therefore easier to harvest.[10] (Another unfortunate example of corporate convenience over God's healing design.) Right when they're closest to being eaten, they're covered in poison. Organic is very important with grains!

There are plenty of wonderful grain-free options out there, too. For example, there are tons of great pasta alternatives on the market these days. Chickpea or lentil pasta (with only a single ingredient) do an incredible job mimicking the taste of conventional pasta. Almond or other nut flour-based baked goods can be just as delicious of a treat. Plus, almonds bring their own nutrients to the table. Brands like Simple Mills (I promise they don't sponsor this book) even have super easy mixes for almond flour brownies and cookies (using coconut sugar as a sweetener). There are even great grain-free pizza crusts out there. Though, at the risk of sounding like a broken record, read the ingredients. Products that are substitutionary in nature (e.g. bread replacement, non-dairy cheese, etc.) often are swimming with nasty additives. Take steps to make your grains or grain-free choices work for your healing!

Dairy

With dairy, the idea here is very similar. Essentially all (and in some states, legally all) milk that is sold in grocery stores is pasteurized. That means that the milk is processed with high heat to kill all the living bacteria in it. This is another late 19th century development that solves one problem but creates a whole mess of others. Yes, the bacteria are dead. But as we've learned, bacteria are not always the enemy. The pasteurization process also deactivates natural enzymes that help our body to break down the lactose.

Not only has pasteurization destroyed most of the nutrients in our milk supply, but the anti-fat trend of the last half-century has, as well. Skim milk might sound healthier, but it is really just an added processing step that removes nourishing fat from the milk (remember, fat isn't inherently evil!). In fact, milk is another example where the processing has removed essentially all the nutrients to the point where conventional sellers need to "fortify" it with added vitamins. That should be an alarm bell to us that the product they're selling has no nutritional value on its own.

Conventional milk also goes through a homogenization process so that we don't have to shake our milk before pouring it into our sugary cereal. It really should be no wonder to us that lactose intolerance is such a rampant issue. Remember, before the 19th century, mankind only drank their milk raw. We have totally destroyed a perfectly healing drink! Raw milk is actually one of the more nutritious things you can put in your body. It hasn't been stripped down to remove the fat. It hasn't been heated up to kill the good bacteria and enzymes. It is alive and full of hard-to-find nutrients like vitamins A and E, magnesium, iodine, and selenium. Many of its nutrients are fat-soluble, which is another reason drinking it whole is important.

We all know that drinking expired pasteurized milk will rot to the point that if you drink it, you'll get sick. But did you know that because of the good bacteria living in it, when raw milk sours, it goes through a natural fermentation that keeps it preserved? I'm not suggesting that you drink sour milk, but I do find it interesting that in milk's natural state, those mighty bacteria continue to do good!

Many people who have trouble digesting pasteurized milk have a much better experience with raw milk. Consider finding a local farm where you can try fresh, A2A2 raw milk from grass-fed jersey cows. A2A2 refers to the protein structure of the milk. Most conventional dairy is from cows which produce A1A2 milk. The A1 protein has been shown to be tougher to digest, plus A2A2 milk helps produce a diverse gut microbiome.[11] Jersey cows are a breed of cows that naturally have the genetics to produce the desired A2A2 milk. If you don't feel comfortable with raw milk, I understand, but I would suggest you cut out as much processed milk from your diet as possible.

As for other dairy products, yogurt and kefir are great options, as they both are fermented and therefore probiotic. Many grocery stores will carry grass-fed, A2A2 milk yogurts. Go for plain yogurts and add in your sweeteners and fruit at home. Honey, granola, açaí powder, and berries (even frozen) are delicious in a bowl of yogurt!

Depending on where you live, you likely can't find raw milk in grocery stores, but you probably can find some raw milk cheeses. Upgrade your cheese game by going for hard cheeses such as sharp cheddar or parmesan that have been aged for at least sixty days. Ideally, these would be made with organic and grass-fed raw milk. Hard cheeses typically have less lactose from the aging process, so they can be easier on our systems, especially if you have a dairy intolerance. Look out for additives in pre-sliced and shredded cheeses. Instead, buy whole blocks of real cheese and slice or shred it yourself.

Nut milks, coconut milk, and other alternatives are readily available these days, but be very careful with a number of shelf-life preservatives, thickening agents (guar or xanthan gum), and sweeteners that are added. If possible, make your nut milks at home or get them from a specialized shop. If you get it from the grocery store, be ready to shake the bottle before you drink. That's far better than unnecessary additives in your alternative milk!

Closing Thoughts

I'll reiterate that I'm not saying you need to cut out all sugar, grains, and dairy from your diet. What I am suggesting is that you should think about the *types* of sugar, grains, and dairy you're eating. Conscientiously consider the least processed, most from-the-earth version of that food and enjoy it in moderation. Or find a replacement that you come to enjoy just as much! Now, if you are in a place of digestive distress, it may be wise, for a time, to severely limit some of these heavy hitters. Remember, we're not trying to adhere to a diet, we are growing an understanding—expanding our knowledge. Don't kick yourself too hard for eating something you know isn't helping you to flourish. Instead, remind yourself that you care more about your long-term health than your short-term pleasure. In time, your desires may just change. Take it one step at a time, in the right direction.

Chapter 14
The Lifestyle

The focus of this book has been about the way that God has designed our bodies to heal themselves. My thesis has been that the right food is the primary avenue of that healing. Alongside that primary avenue, there are secondary ones as well. There are so many life practices that can support your body in healing. I want to spend a little bit of time here diving into some of the practices that, alongside the right foods, can make a real mark in your health journey.

Knowledge Is Power

I'll start by repeating my plea from a couple chapters ago: use your head. It's worth mentioning again here but from a bit of a different perspective. One of the most powerful practices you can put in place is growing in your knowledge of how the body works, what it thrives on, and what to do to support it. Read some books (good job getting this deep into my book), listen to some podcasts, watch a documentary, or talk to a local farmer. There is a growing library of resources that are both fascinating and practical for everyday life. Open up your world to truly life-changing information. It is a better use of your time than another football game or streaming show.

The more you can chew on (pun intended), the more you can begin to put pieces together. Maybe you start to catch onto certain themes from various sources. Maybe you hear conflicting viewpoints and want to find the truth. Maybe you learn something that stretches your mind and challenges your status quo. These are good things. Challenge your mind to help your body.

Here are a few of the most potent and informative resources that I've run across. By the way, none of these people paid me to put these on this list.

Books

- *Ancient Remedies* by Dr. Josh Axe
- *Breaking the Vicious Cycle* by Elaine Gloria Gottschall (a deep dive into the specific carb diet, which Haley used in her healing journey)
- *Non-Toxic* by Drs. Aly Cohen and Frederick von Saal
- *Nourishing Traditions* by Sally Fallon
- *Restoring Your Digestive Health* by Jordan Rubin
- *Food Healed Me* and cookbooks by Danielle Walker
- *The Mind-Gut Connection* by Dr. Emeran Mayer
- *Folks, This Ain't Normal* by Joel Salatin
- *The End of Craving* by Mark Schatzker

Podcasts & Other Resources

- *Ancient Health* Podcast by Dr. Josh Axe

- *The Doctor's Farmacy* Podcast by Dr. Mark Hyman

- *Wise Traditions* Podcast by Hilda Gore

- *Be Organic* Podcast by Kat and Landon Eckles

- *The Art of Manliness* Podcast by Brett and Kate McKay, specifically: Episodes 754, 852, 862, 866, and other health-oriented episodes

- *Food, Inc.* Documentary directed by Robert Kenner

- Healthline.com

- The references in the back of this book

Those are obviously not comprehensive lists of resources. They are just a starting place. Find what piques your interest and invest some real time into understanding your body better. Learn about how it works, why certain things affect us in certain ways, how our current environment has deteriorated our health, and more. Get interested and get into it!

Community

Our ancestors, the early church, heck—even our great-grandparents lived in what would be considered a radical community today. They supported each other, served each other, and fed each other. If you are going to be consistent long-term in living out a healing lifestyle, you need to do it in community. That may mean just one other person, or it may mean a full support system. Maybe it's your spouse, a roommate, your kids, a group of friends, or even the church. For example, how powerful would it be if instead of Papa John's at every church youth group event, we worked together to provide nourishing, real food to our kids?

If you try to lone wolf it, you're likely destined to end up right back where you started. This is especially important at home. That is where support or resistance may make or break a healing lifestyle. If your spouse (or kids or roommate) doesn't initially want to support this kind of lifestyle, help them understand *why* it matters, rather than forcing the change. Whoever your community ends up being, commit to helping each other in accountability, consistency, and enjoyment of healing food. Thank God together for the healing food He perfectly designed for us. Get excited to try new things together.

Prioritize Cooking at Home

If you want to improve the quality of foods that you're eating, you need to know exactly what it is you're actually eating. The only way to really do that is to prioritize cooking at home. When you're eating out, even when you go somewhere that you consider "healthy," you never truly know the full ins and outs of your meal. For example, while Chipotle is delicious and typically is on the more conscientious side when it comes to selecting ingredients, they also use rice bran oil, sunflower seed oil, and canola oil across many of their products. Even Chipotle's steak (which could simply be cooked in its own fat) is cooked in sunflower oil.[1] These are each highly processed, seed-based oils full of polyunsaturated fat, which quickly decompose in our bodies. Unfortunately, in today's world, it is so hard to find true healing food at a restaurant.

What's the solution? Become a chef! I'm kidding, kind of. Make it your goal to cook up a majority of your meals. Plan ahead enough to have leftovers for lunch the next day. Carve out time in your schedule, at least a few times a week, to be in the kitchen. Doing this forces you to slow your day down, take forty-five minutes to breathe, and even exercise some creative muscles.

Avoid using the microwave. That isn't true cooking; rather, it's a pitfall from our idolization of convenience. It doesn't add healing potential (or taste, for that matter) to God's design for our food.

Maybe you don't love cooking. Or maybe you don't think you know how. Trust me, it really isn't as hard as it seems. You may start out re-reading recipes fifteen times and getting frustrated at the blog post in front of every online recipe. But consistency in the kitchen also leads to comfortability. Once you do it enough, you'll start getting the hang of it. You'll look less at recipes and more at the fridge with the endless possibilities of glorious flavor and healing potential! I've been personally shocked at how many seemingly difficult recipes are really quite simple. For example, making hummus, granola, yogurt, fermented foods, or bone broth may seem unattainable but, in reality, they are quite simple, delicious, and economical. Reducing the quantity of meals eaten at a restaurant is one of the easiest ways to make a healing lifestyle cost-effective.

Economical Healing

Often, money is cited as the primary reason for many people to not pursue a healing lifestyle. Yes, it's true that a bag of organic granola costs more than a box of Frosted Flakes, but the mindset of "Healthy food is too expensive" is too simplistic to be a valid excuse. For starters, as we've discussed earlier in this book, organic isn't a newfangled fad; it's a return to the way the human race grew its food for millennia. On the contrary, the too-good-to-be-true prices of fast food and over-processed foods are actually just that: too good to be true. Those prices would not even be possible without the insane policies of corn and soybean subsidies. The mindset shouldn't be "Healthy food is too expensive" but rather "Unhealthy food is too cheap"! And that's saying nothing of the long-term savings you'll have in medical costs by avoiding the innumerable diseases caused by consistently damaging eating. Living a healing lifestyle doesn't just include food costs, it saves on healthcare costs!

Let's say you conceptually agree with that, but on some level, when the rubber meets the road, you've only got so much money and you've got to decide where to spend it. I don't know your specific situation, but I do know this: there is a path forward for you, no matter what your budget looks like. What we prioritize, we'll make space for, so I urge you to make a healing lifestyle a priority. It is truly one of the most important things you can spend your money on. It's an investment in you and your family's future.

Some practical possibilities include focusing on the "Dirty Dozen" (as mentioned in Chapter 12) for buying organic. These are the crops which are most sprayed with pesticides, and therefore the organic versions give you the most healing bang for your buck. For the latest version head to: *www.ewg.org/foodnews/dirty-dozen.php*.

Rather than finding the "healthy" replacement for boxed and bagged foods (these are usually quite pricey), focus on buying unprocessed, whole foods. Typically, hardier vegetables like carrots, sweet potatoes, squash (butternut, spaghetti, or acorn), and beets tend to be on the cheaper side per pound and last longer. Reduce as much waste as you can. That certainly includes not letting your produce go bad. But it also means eating more parts of your produce. For example, many root vegetables (beets, carrots, turnips, etc.) also have edible dark leafy greens—two for one!

The freezer is also your friend for preventing spoilage. Before letting things go bad, you can freeze fruit, dark leafy greens, and avocados for smoothies. You can even buy some of your produce frozen, which can often be cheaper (due to low risk of spoilage for the seller). Frozen veggies (like cauliflower rice and green peas) taste great as add-ins for stir fries or soups. However, be aware that frozen veggies may not be as appetizing as a stand-alone side (no thank you, mushy green beans). Frozen bone broth also keeps very well.

Buying local and in-season is often cheaper than buying organic produce at the grocery store because of the reduced supply chain costs incurred when shipping the product halfway around the world. You could join a Community Supported Agriculture (CSA) farm to cut out the middleman and therefore some expense. Basically, with a CSA you buy a share of the produce that farm grows and pick it up straight from the farmer.

Wisdom in serving sizes is helpful as well. In other words, you don't need to feel stuffed after every meal. Limiting snacking can quickly cut down on costs, too. Haley and I find we spend less money if we shop more at the farmer's market because we aren't drawn towards the colorful marketing of the snack aisle at the grocery store. Of course, leftovers are a money saver. You can make dinners large enough for a couple nights that week, then make a large batch lunch option like organic rotisserie chickens, soups, or quinoa bowls, which will last a few servings. Check out the Appendix for some recipe ideas.

Some creativity in meals can also save you some dough. Mix and match things that you have on hand instead of buying items for a specific recipe. This will become more of a possibility the more you cook at home because you'll have staples in stock and know what flavors you enjoy together. Maybe you have leftover quinoa, black beans, broccoli, pesto, and chicken from various meals—throw them together and all of a sudden you have something new. You may find you like some combos you weren't expecting. And obviously, the less wasted food the better for the wallet.

Get your food as whole as possible, not just for nutrients but for economics. Buy a whole chicken instead of just the boneless, skinless breasts. Or buy the whole fruit instead of pre-sliced. The less processing it has to go through, the cheaper it is due to lower labor costs. By buying whole, you can prevent waste and maximize your dollar. For example, you can eat the chicken breasts for one meal, then chop up the dark meat for tacos, and save the bones for broth which turns into a hearty soup. With the bones of two chickens (both of which you have eaten all the meat from), you can make four quarts of the highest quality bone broth, which would cost you more than $50 at the grocery store from what was otherwise scraps. Talk about economical!

Other foods are just plain cheap, even the high-quality versions. You can buy a couple boxes of organic chickpeas for something like

$2.50. Then you can make a boatload of additive-free hummus for a fraction of the price you'd be paying for it pre-made. Organic steel-cut oats are very affordable, and a single cup will typically make 3-4 servings for breakfasts. Organic grass-fed A2A2 yogurt may be more than Yoplait, but if you buy it in a larger container rather than single serving cups, it is still a great deal. These are typically around $5 and will offer you plenty of healthy snack or breakfast servings. Plus, if you buy it plain, it not only is free of added sugar, but you can also change up the flavors. Pro tip: try a dessert yogurt with cacao powder, peanut butter, and maple syrup. You'll thank me later.

There are solutions if you're willing to search for them. Eventually, the economics will follow the demand. I mean, Wal-Mart sells organic food now, for Pete's sake. That didn't happen out of their altruistic desire to see you be happier and healthier. It's because they know people want to buy those products. As that happens more often, prices decline, volume increases, and everyone has better access to real, whole foods.

Fasting

Fasting is the practice of skipping meals on purpose for a specific reason. If you're like me, the first thing that comes to mind when fasting is mentioned is a spiritual experience. God didn't design the different parts of our being to be siloed. Our spiritual and our physical lives are intertwined. While there are innumerable spiritual benefits to fasting, there are also significant physical ones, as well. Basically, fasting gives your body a breather. Our gut isn't designed to be digesting food 24/7, which is what the typical Western diet forces it to do. Think about your gut as a business owner who can never get around to growing the business because they're too laser focused on working the cash register. Fasting gives your gut a chance to pause the operational work of digestion to focus on the strategic work of healing.

There are some astounding stories out there about folks who suffered from chronic diseases, and fasting was their primary source of healing. This is due, in part, because when our body doesn't have food to metabolize into energy, it reverts to using fat stores instead. This produces a compound called a ketone in your liver. Healthy cells can use ketones as fuel instead of our normal fuel (glucose), but unhealthy cells don't have that ability due to their weak mitochondria.[2] Basically, fasting simultaneously starves unhealthy cells and feeds healthy ones! It may be uncomfortable or unfamiliar, but it's a potent healing tool.

There are lots of different ways to fast. It may be as simple as intentionally skipping a meal while continuing to drink lots of water. You could also try a juice cleanse, which has the advantage of getting nutrients from organic green juices without your gut needing to digest anything. Or perhaps you try a bone broth fast, which gives you a bit more of a satiated feeling (due to its higher protein content) while packing a powerful healing punch. Start small and work your way up, in terms of the length of the fast. Try a meal and see how you feel, then make it a day before jumping to anything longer. Be consistent in fasting at least once a month, even just a single meal. Make this restful practice part of your ordinary routine, not an outlier. Then you will also be prepared for a longer fast if you're feeling your gut have any major issues. A fast can be one of your first lines of defense in combating dangerous gut inflammation. With all of that said, please don't stop eating only to lose weight. Healing and weight loss are not the same thing. In fact, weight loss can be distinctly unhealthy. If you struggle with an eating disorder, fasting may not be the best choice for you at the moment.

Micronutrients

Micronutrients are the vitamins and minerals that our bodies use to support cell growth, immune response, energy production, and many other vital bodily functions. These include commonly known vitamins such as vitamin C and lesser-known micronutrients like selenium. The truth is that many of us are likely deficient in some of these micronutrients, which contributes to many health concerns. It often takes an intentional effort to maintain a robust range of these micronutrients to support our bodies.

Supplements (also known as "vitamins") are a common way of trying to remedy this situation. They are typically capsules of isolated micronutrients. Supplements can certainly be helpful, but only if they are used (as the name suggests) to *supplement* a diet that gives you most of what you need nutrition-wise. Your body can only absorb so much from a pill. The goal should be to get a vast majority of your micronutrients from the food itself. If you know (via a blood test) or suspect that you are deficient in a certain area, then supplements may be a great addition. Most of us are likely deficient in vitamin B, vitamin D, zinc, and omega-3 fatty acids, so if you're looking to supplement, those may be a good place to start.

If I could only recommend one type of supplement, it would be a probiotic. Probiotic supplements support the microbiome by filling it with helpful bacteria. Along with probiotics, digestive enzymes can support gut health, especially if you're facing an active digestive crisis. If you are looking for personalized direction on a supplement routine, consider finding a local naturopathic doctor. These holistic doctors can test to identify what deficiencies you may be battling and support you in selecting the right kind and quantity of supplements.

When it comes to supplements, the whole food idea is still in place. These supplements don't necessarily have to look like pills. They could be powders, juices, or in liquid drops. Find quality supplements that use actual foods in their makeup (otherwise you might be paying for synthetic versions of the micronutrient). For example, elderberry or certain species of mushrooms can be found in supplement form for immune boosting. Dehydrated grass-fed beef liver capsules are a great source of vitamins A and B. Curcumin, the potent anti-inflammatory active ingredient of turmeric, can be found in supplement form. You can even use herbal teas as a supplement of sorts. These teas provide your body with healing herbs like milk thistle and ashwagandha. Of course, never forget to read the ingredient label for additives; they can be found in supplements as much as anywhere else.

The table on the next page is a *starting place* for where to find some of the important micronutrients directly from whole foods. Of course, it is not an exhaustive list of where these nutrients are found. Try to keep your food selections varied across this table to consistently get each of these vital micronutrients. If there is a micronutrient in this table that you feel you cannot consistently get through food, perhaps consider a supplement form of that nutrient.

Micronutrient	Sources
Vitamin A	Grass-Fed Beef Liver, Raw Milk, Eggs, Açaí
Vitamin B	Grass-Fed Beef Liver, Salmon, Spirulina
Vitamin C	Citrus Fruits, Broccoli, Camu Camu
Vitamin D	Sunlight, Salmon, Grass-Fed Beef Liver
Vitamin E	Almonds, Peanuts, Hazelnuts
Vitamin K	Kale, Spinach, Brussel Sprouts
Calcium	Raw Milk, Raw Cheese
Magnesium	Almonds, Peanuts, Raw Milk
Zinc	Grass-Fed Beef, Chicken
Selenium	Brazil Nuts, Grass-Fed Beef Liver
Manganese	Lentils, Steel-Cut Oats, Flaxseed
Iodine	Grass-Fed Beef Liver, Raw Milk, Eggs
Probiotics	Grass-Fed Yogurt, Sauerkraut, Kombucha
Omega-3 Fatty Acids	Salmon, Chia Seeds, Flaxseed

Move

Aside from diet, the thing that everyone knows is good for you, but most of us don't really want to do is exercise. I don't believe you'll ever be able to work out enough to overcome a terrible diet. In fact, trying to outwork your diet is really a profound misunderstanding of the purpose of exercise. We weren't designed for diet and exercise to be on opposite ends of the bodily scales, hoping that our exercise outweighs our food intake. Instead, we were designed for movement and diet to work together toward our holistic health.

Movement is simply foundational to our health. Here are just a few benefits: movement boosts metabolism, improves sleep, protects your heart, strengthens your bones, and even improves your mental health. Your body will be better suited to digest all the healing foods you are now feeding it if you're also moving!

We have become an increasingly sedentary society, which has certainly been a factor in the massive decline in our collective health. Find ways to incorporate consistent movement into your daily life. Do it outside if you can. Get more sunlight in your life, especially in the morning. Breathe in fresh air. During long stretches of sedentary time, think of ways to move. Maybe you can take a walk during a meeting you're only listening to. Or, if you work from home, try a few yoga stretches a couple times during the workday. Get up and move at least once every hour.

When you want a more intense workout, pair cardio with strength training. Don't overdo it on one or the other. The combination of the two produces a *temporary* inflammation in our body, which actually trains our body to be able to combat dangerous *chronic* inflammation. That said, be careful not to set goals that will end up either crushing your motivation or laying unnecessary guilt on yourself. It's not about how hard you push yourself. It's not even about burning calories or PRs. You'll get the most benefit by keeping your body moving consistently and pairing that with food that will support your flourishing.

Rest

Alongside movement, find rhythms of rest in your life. Detox not just from foods that harm but from schedules that do their fair share of damage. Keep your phone out of your room at night (buy a real alarm clock if you need to). Turn off ninety percent of the notifications on your phone (is it *really* imperative that you get a push notification the moment the Red Sox score a run?). Read more books. Take a break from social media or YouTube. Wake up early and pray. Keep a journal. Take a real sabbath. If God rested, so can you. In fact, you absolutely need to, or your health will come tumbling down. It is astounding how many diseases even a conventional, Western doctor will tell you are triggered, if not outright caused, by stress.

Rest doesn't happen by accident. Make room for it in your life. But don't buy cheap rest. Hours of TV or staring at your phone don't bring you real rest. Plan a day where you have no plan and no technology and see what happens. It may start out feeling boring, but by the end of it you'll be ready to take on the world. The ironic thing is that we are more able and willing to be productive in our everyday lives if we take a moment to stop them and rest.

The most obvious form of rest that I didn't mention is sleep. Take sleep seriously. Our world degrades the importance of it. We like to hype up efficiency, ultra-productivity, and burning the candle at both ends. Don't give into that lie. Sleeping can be medicine for both your body and your soul. Essentially, your body is always either working or healing. It is hard-pressed to do both. Give your body uninterrupted healing time.

Some of the key healing factors of sleep include its relationship with hormone production and heart health. During sleep, your body becomes more sensitive to insulin, supporting healthy blood sugar levels. On top of that, growth hormone is released, which empowers the repair of cells. Your heart rate slows and your blood pressure drops, giving your cardiovascular system a break.[3] Improved sleep can also have a serious effect on lowering stress, and lowering stress can then have a powerful effect on physical and mental flourishing.

Prepare yourself to sleep. Dim the lights and stay away from screens for an hour before bed. Drink a warm mug of chamomile tea. Read a few pages of a book. Don't just expect your body to sleep when you want it to. Let it know that it's time to slow down and rest.

Two other rest-adjacent practices you can implement are massages and sweating it out in an infrared sauna. I bet you can handle those prescriptions. Massages are both a physical and mental break. They loosen your knots *and* force you to be silent for a whole hour. Crazy. The infrared sauna also gives you some time alone (or with a partner) to rest, get away from technology, and literally sweat out toxins. Sweating is the body's ancient detox method. It's one of the reasons that movement is so important. But finding alternative methods of sweating it out, like the sauna, can be really effective, too. Sweating (via the sauna or exercise) can be particularly effective in detoxing heavy metals from your body.[4]

Home Products

As you get deeper into the healing lifestyle, I can almost guarantee that you will want to expand the boundaries. Beauty products are a black hole of nasty additives and applying them directly to your skin every day will not end well. Similarly, cleaning products are often the furthest thing from clean. Over-the-counter medications can cause liver and other organ damage. You can't change everything at once, but start thinking about what chemicals go in, on, or around your body every day and consider natural alternatives.

For beauty products, start by avoiding polyethylene glycols (PEGs), which may be a human carcinogen.[5] Aluminum is a common ingredient in antiperspirant and can build up in your body after repeated usage. For cleaning products, avoid artificial fragrances and harsh chemicals. If you'd need to call poison control if you swallowed it, then why do we want to clean our counters with it? Good ol' baking soda and vinegar are great for more than just your 5th grade papier mâché volcanoes; they also make a powerful cleaning combo. Some essential oils (like clove) also have antiviral properties and therefore act as a powerful all-purpose cleaner when mixed with water.

For medications, make it your goal to avoid using medicines that you don't actually need. Popping acetaminophen or a decongestant may be the norm, but the more you use them, the more risk you're at of them causing serious organ damage. Consider natural options like a neti-pot (for sinus clearing with just water and salt), an Epsom salt bath (for sore joints and muscles), or raw honey (as an antibacterial ointment for wounds). These natural remedies may seem strange at first, but I bet you'll find them more effective than you expect. For example, one study found that "honey has almost equal or slightly superior effects when compared with conventional treatments for acute wounds and superficial partial thickness burns."[6] God designed His creation to support us in healing!

Closing Thoughts

This chapter has been a 30,000-foot view of many *huge* topics. Each of them could be a book on their own. If you need personalized support living out this healing design, consider finding a local naturopathic doctor. These are trained medical professionals who will consider your holistic health and natural remedies rather than a pharmaceutical route. They may point you to a chiropractor or an acupuncturist. Or they can run tests on your hormone and micro-nutrient levels. Their knowledge and personalized method can be exactly what you need if you're fighting an active battle toward healing.

None of us will ever live a perfectly non-toxic life as long as we're also living relatively ordinary American lives. And that's okay. We're not aiming for perfection, rather for flourishing habits. It's about what your "normal" is. Don't get bogged down with where you're starting but focus on where you're heading. Move in the right direction when it comes to living in God's healing design. Help your body to combat the toxins that constantly surround us, rather than fall prey to them. Pick one of these practices and try it. Give it time and see how your body reacts to it. Then pick a new one to add in. Take it one step at a time, in the right direction. You can do it!

Conclusion
More Than Physical

I'll conclude this book with an echo of the conclusion to Part I. That's because Part I is my favorite. It's the part that changed our lives. Part II is the unfortunate reality that forced the need for this book. The idea that we've both personally and culturally corrupted God's good design for food and healing is vital to grasp, but it's not fun. And Part III just scratches the surface of the outflowing implications and applications for our lives. But Part I is all about hope, possibility, faith, and healing.

It is a paradigm shift.

Once you grasp the idea that God not only designed your body with the ability to heal, but He provided the ways and means to get there, all of a sudden, the seemingly crushing weight of physical decay loses its power.

All of a sudden, you don't need to identify yourself by your disease.

All of a sudden, you have a medicine that builds you up instead of tears you down.

All of a sudden, you're in tune with your body instead of battling against it.

This paradigm shift isn't an isolated incident. It is actually a side effect of God's big story. It's not just our food and healing that is marred by sin. Every aspect of our lives has been corrupted in a way that prevented us from living out our God-given design. In fact, mankind wholly rejected that design and God Himself. But God, in His unimaginable grace, sent His Son to Earth. Jesus lived the sinless life that we couldn't. He died the condemned death that we deserved. And if we repent of our rejection of Him and believe that Jesus is the savior we need, we can be reunited with God and His design in every aspect of life.

God tells humanity a story of hope, possibility, faith, and healing. And that healing is far more than just a physical healing. It is one that touches all parts of us. In what Jesus called the greatest commandment, He tells us:

> "And you shall love the Lord your God with all your heart and with all your soul and with all your mind and with all your strength."
>
> MARK 12:30

Our heart, soul, mind, and strength make up who we are as persons. God has a healing path for each part of our being. The healing of our strength (the physical part) is probably what started you on this journey. It did for Haley and me. But I guarantee it's not the best part of the journey. The healing of our mind (the mental part) and our heart (the emotional part) is an astoundingly beautiful effect of living in God's good design. We learned that as we walk in God's design for our strength by eating the food that God designed, our mind and our heart flourish, too. The miraculous gut microbiome is the axis point of our strength, our mind, and our heart.

All of this ultimately leads to our soul (the spiritual part). Once we see God's good design in one aspect of our lives, our eyes begin to be opened to His design in *every* aspect of our lives. We start to believe more and more every day that all of what He says is *actually true*. He *really has* invited us into His family and called us by name. That motivates us to fight to live in His design more fully. Our souls are nourished along with our bodies.

God has a healing path for our whole self. That healing is for us, yes. But it's also for Him. As Jesus said in Mark 12:30, each of these aspects of our being can be a part of loving the Lord our God. One of the ways we obey the command to love Him is by trusting in and walking in His design. That expression of our love brings God glory. As we seek after and walk in His good design for our food, our healing, and our physical flourishing, we can bring the God of the universe glory. Isn't that incredible?

Our God has always been a healer. Since you were created in His image, you are...

Designed to Heal

Appendix
Kitchen Tools

Kitchens can get cluttered fast with bulky appliances you never use. These are some of our favorite powerhouses that are actually worth keeping around:

- **Instant Pot**: There are tons of uses, but I typically use it for yogurt, bone broth, chili, beans/lentils, applesauce, and cooking whole chickens.

- **Vitamix**: You can't go wrong with these super powerful blenders. They're great for smoothies, hummus, pesto, and soups, among many other things. Some recipes do work better with a food processor, but you can make a Vitamix work in most scenarios.

- **Le Creuset Dutch Oven**: These are great for soups, roasting meat, and sautéing veggies.

- **Cast Iron Skillet**: I love the versatility and simplicity of the cast iron. I will also use ceramic and stainless-steel skillets, but avoid non-stick pans, which often have chemical coatings that can leach into your food. Plus, if you're using the right fats, any pan is non-stick!

- **Mason Jars**: These classics are great for storage and canning. In general, try to avoid plastic storage and replace it with glass. Mason jars come in a variety of sizes up to a full gallon. Wide-mouth versions are ideal for fermentation.

- **Fermentation Lid**: Well, it's in the name, but these handy lids (which attach to mason jars) prevent mold from growing by locking out oxygen during the fermentation process.

- **Mortar & Pestle**: Simple, manual, elegant. These are great for getting your elbow grease into sauces, spices, and dressings. The first salad dressing in the *Recipes* section of this appendix is a great example of what you can make with a mortar and pestle.

- **Chemex Pour Over**: Personally, I believe this is the way to make real coffee. Like the mortar and pestle, I love that there are no buttons, no plug-ins, just fresh ground coffee beans and hot water.

- **Loose Leaf Tea Infuser**: Instead of store-bought tea bags, find a local organic farm or shop who produces their own loose-leaf teas. As a bonus, you can reuse loose leaf tea for multiple cups. Astragalus and ginger are great immune-boosting herbal teas. Chamomile and tulsi can be effective at calming. Slippery elm and marshmallow root are great gut-supporting options.

Brands We Love

Of course, most of our foods should be whole foods in their natural form, but when the time comes for a convenient packaged food, there are some great options! Below is a list of some of our favorite brands we've discovered over the years:

- **Simple Mills**: You may have guessed this one, but when it comes to boxed foods, it doesn't get much better than them. They have simple, mostly organic ingredients and delicious snacks anyone would enjoy.

- **Siete Foods**: They make a grain-free, seed-oil-free tortilla chip that is out of this world.

- **LesserEvil**: Another solid snack brand that uses all organic and simple ingredients. The Paleo Puffs and Sun Poppers are easy treats. Pro-tip: grab a bag of Sun Poppers for a movie; it's cheaper and dramatically better for you than movie theater popcorn.

- **Skout Organic Bars**: Finding a decent protein bar for a quick snack is tough, but Skout does it well with simple and organic ingredients.

- **Hu Kitchen**: High-quality organic baking and snacking chocolate sweetened with coconut sugar and no added emulsifiers.

- **Evolved Chocolate**: We are such big chocolate fans, I had to mention a second amazing option. Organic cacao-based chocolate bars with simple, delicious fillings. Yum.

- **Kettle & Fire**: The tastiest, long-simmered bone broths without the need to add "natural chicken flavor" like most brands do.

- **Primal Kitchen**: When it comes to condiments and sauces, it doesn't get much better than Primal Kitchen unless you make it yourself.

- **Ancient Nutrition**: There are so many shady supplement companies out there, so it's important to find one you trust. Ancient Nutrition does an awesome job using real foods for their vitamins and minerals while also minimizing additives.

- **Purity Coffee**: Coffee is a heavily sprayed crop, so organic is very important. Purity is not only organic, but it tests for mold and other toxins. It also roasts to a specific point which maximizes antioxidants. Plus, it just tastes incredible.

Recipes (Sort Of)

I said in the introduction that this is not a cookbook. That hasn't changed, but I thought it could be helpful to provide some instructions for a few staples of a healing diet. With that being said, these are less recipes and more general processes. What I hope you gain from this appendix is a view into the thought process of making a meal. Every meal you make at home grows your understanding of flavors and methods that work well together. Yes, some dishes take more precision than others, but the vast majority of cooking is practice, feel, creativity, and rhythm. Cooking really is more of an art than a science. Have fun, make mistakes, enjoy yourself!

Meals and Sides

Roasted Veggies

I mentioned this one earlier in the book, but it's so foundational that it's worth repeating. Most veggies are delicious roasted. I typically will dump them in a big mixing bowl, pour on a solid dose of olive oil, and throw them in a 385°F oven for about 15 minutes. Check them and see if they've started to crisp up (or for denser veggies, soften up). If not, go a few more minutes. This works great for green beans, broccoli, brussels sprouts, butternut squash, beets, carrots, potatoes, sweet potatoes, cauliflower, etc. Some may require an extra step or two, such as peeling or chopping, but generally it all works the same. If you sauté, try using some high-quality animal fats like grass-fed butter or tallow. These saturated fats have higher smoke points and are therefore safer for high-heat cooking.

Whole Chicken

Cooking the whole bird limits waste, is helpful for meal prep, and is very economical. Start by patting dry your bird and seasoning it with any variety of herbs and spices (basil, oregano, garlic, and thyme are great options). Put a small layer of water in your Instant Pot, set up the trivet, and lay the chicken breast-side up. Cook on high pressure for about 5 minutes per pound, so usually around 15-20 minutes. You can broil it for a minute or two to crisp the skin after it's done cooking. A Dutch oven can be used to roast the chicken if you don't have an Instant Pot. Typically, night one I'll carve the breasts and enjoy them fresh. Then I'll remove the thigh and leg quarters for two more servings. The rest of the meat you can get off the bones with your hands and chop up for pizza, tacos, or other shredded meat meals. But save those bones!

Bone Broth

This massively healing, anti-inflammatory food is so simple to make at home in the Instant Pot. I haven't made it without one, but I imagine it is also quite simple, though it takes much longer. With the Instant Pot, essentially all you do is put all the ingredients in the pot, fill near to the max line with filtered water, and put on high pressure for 4 hours. Then, strain and store (refrigerate or freeze). As for what those ingredients are, the most important one is (obviously) the bones themselves. You'll need the bones from two chickens. The easiest option is to make whole chickens and save the bones. If you don't make them quickly enough, freeze the first set until you make the second. Once you have two chickens' worth of bones, use them as your primary ingredient in the broth. Add a couple teaspoons of apple cider vinegar and some salt, and that's all you really need.

Other great add-ins for health and/or flavor include mushrooms, astragalus, cinnamon sticks, peppercorns, ginger, turmeric, and bay leaf. You can also add four or five chicken feet for a more gelatinous broth, which is good for gut health.

Chicken Soup

Now that you know how to make a whole chicken and homemade bone broth, you can put it all together in a soup! The dark meat can be shredded up and used as the protein. Organic chicken sausage is another great option. Most soups we make are simply a combination of whatever leftovers are in the fridge. Start by sautéing veggies like bell pepper, carrot, onion, garlic, and/or celery in a large pot or Dutch oven (if you're using chicken sausage, throw it in there too). Once everything is smelling good, add in enough chicken broth to fill the soup and let it simmer for approximately 15 minutes. Add in some herbs and spices like turmeric, paprika, cumin, oregano, or basil. Finally, add in some frozen cauliflower rice and spinach, if you like. Soup is really just an easy way to mix and match leftovers into a cohesive meal—don't overthink it!

Quinoa Bowls

Quinoa is not technically a grain (rather it's a seed), but it has the fiber and protein to make a great base for a meal. Use two parts water to one part dry quinoa, simply boiling it until the water is absorbed. It is now the perfect canvas for flavor, as it has very little itself. Season generously! As for the rest of the bowl, use the roasted veggies or shredded chicken from above. Ground salmon, pork, or grass-fed beef are all great options. Essentially quinoa + protein + veggies + spices = filling and delicious meal.

Salad Dressing

Store-bought salad dressings are full of seed-based oils, sugar, and additives. Make it at home instead! Here are two quick, easy options. First, chop or smash two cloves of garlic, pour in a few tablespoons of olive oil, add a couple squirts of stone-ground mustard, and fresh-grated raw parmesan cheese. Mix that all together and it makes any salad worth eating. The second option is even easier: mix olive oil and a cooking vinegar (like apple cider, balsamic, or red wine vinegar) together. It should be mostly oil with enough vinegar for a nice bite. If you can find a local shrub producer, that is even better. Shrubs are fruit-infused apple cider vinegars, and they're delicious!

Applesauce

If you have an Instant Pot, homemade applesauce is an absolute must! It is about as easy as any recipe can be. Simply peel and core about six red apples and six green apples. Chop them into chunks (they don't need to be too small). Put those in your Instant Pot and cover with about a cup of water. Sprinkle some cinnamon on top and stir to combine. Then set on high pressure for eight minutes. Once it's done, you'll want to let it naturally release pressure or else you'll have apples spraying out of your release valve! Once the pressure is released, stir until it's smooth and enjoy it hot or cold.

Sauces and Toppings

Sauerkraut/Fermented Veggies

I talked earlier about the significant benefits of fermented veggies like sauerkraut. They are quite simple to make at home, though they do teach you a lesson in patience! Essentially, you need a veggie, water, salt, and time. Using sauerkraut as the example, you start by chopping a cabbage up into thin strips. Then add about 2-2.5% of the weight of the cabbage in salt. Massage the salt into the cabbage and the salt will pull the water right out of the veggie, creating a natural brine. Let it sit for about 10 minutes, then pack both the cabbage and the brine tight in a mason jar. The key here is to not let any cabbage touch the air. If it's under the brine, it won't grow mold, but above the brine it's at risk. This is where the fermentation lid comes in handy. As the fermenting bacteria create carbon dioxide, that pushes the oxygen out and the lid prevents it from coming back in, effectively preventing mold (which needs oxygen). Let it ferment at room temperature for about three weeks, just keeping an eye out for anything weird growing. Otherwise, it should finish up with a sour and tangy flavor and is a great topping on sandwiches, burgers, tacos, salads, and more!

Hummus

I'll let you find a recipe for the exact measurements for hummus, but I thought it was worth mentioning here because it is just so easy and cost-effective to make at home. It was one of those things I never even realized you could make at home. Then once I tried, I was shocked at how much better it was than store-bought. Essentially, you need chickpeas (or garbanzo beans—which are the same thing, who knew?), tahini (which is basically sesame seed butter), olive oil, garlic, cumin, and salt. Blend these ingredients up until they're smooth, and deliciousness awaits.

Pesto

Similar to hummus, pesto is incredibly simple and can be made by essentially dumping all the ingredients into a Vitamix and hitting blend. Typically, pesto consists of fresh basil, olive oil, (raw) parmesan cheese, pine nuts, and garlic. You can also get creative with other leafy greens to supplement the basil. Pesto is great as pizza sauce, pasta sauce, or just slathering on chicken.

Breakfast

Yogurt

This is one that I assumed was so difficult that I could never make it at home...until I tried! Admittedly, having an Instant Pot (or some other yogurt maker) certainly makes things easier, but there are DIY versions with a cooler and heat packs, if you're really feeling creative. Essentially, yogurt is fermented milk. That means you need high-quality milk and some bacteria. And that's it; those are the ingredients! For milk, I use raw milk from a local farmer. Even if it's not raw, look for the A2A2, minimally processed, whole milk. I haven't tried this with alternative milks, but I imagine it is much more delicate of a process. As for the bacteria, the easiest option is simply to mix in a spoonful of high-quality store-bought yogurt. The probiotic starter you're looking for is the "Live Active Cultures" listed on the store-bought yogurt's ingredient list. Use a half gallon of milk with a couple spoonfuls of the probiotic starter and put the Instant Pot on the yogurt setting for 8-12 hours. The yogurt setting essentially keeps the temperature around 110°F, which is exactly the temperature at which the probiotics like to multiply. After the incubation period, the yogurt should be formed and not liquidy. Whisk it up to get the right texture, or you can strain in a cheesecloth if you want a thicker, Greek style.

Frittata

If you don't know what a frittata is, don't fret. Just think of a quiche without a crust. This is one dish where a cast iron skillet comes in handy. Crack five eggs into a bowl, whisk them up, and mix in your spices of choice (salt, pepper, oregano, basil, etc.). Sauté up some veggies in the cast iron skillet. Really any will do, but some classic options include peppers, onions, spinach, or mushrooms. Once the veggies are ready, pour the eggs into the skillet and throw it into the oven at 400°F for 15 to 20 minutes. Voilà! You look like a brunch expert.

Overnight Oats

I mentioned earlier in the book that oats can be one of the most nutritious grains out there. I also mentioned that steel-cut oats are the least processed version. Well, they also are the least convenient to make, which (I imagine) is exactly why they are the least common. Overnight oats are the solution to that. Add four parts water to one part steel-cut oats to a pot and bring to a boil for only one minute. This prepares the oats to soak in water overnight. Then cover and throw in the fridge until the morning. This not only dramatically reduces necessary cook time, but it also helps our bodies flourish. Soaking grains and seeds help to remove anti-nutrients that can be present. It also makes them easier to digest. I also tend to find that this method makes the oats last for more servings, too. All around wins! Okay, now that it's the morning, simply put the pot back on the burner, bring to a boil, and simmer for about 10 minutes or whenever it reaches a good consistency. Enjoy!

Chia Pudding

The last recipe I'll share is more unique, but it's a great one. Chia pudding is a super easy, yogurt-like breakfast (or snack) option. Into a mason jar, pour a cup of the milk of your choice (dairy or otherwise), four tablespoons of chia seeds, a quick pour of maple syrup, and a splash of vanilla extract. Close the mason jar and shake. Let it sit a few minutes and you'll notice the chia seeds separating. Repeat the shaking process a couple times and after a few minutes, the mixture will start to congeal. At that point, throw it in the fridge and it'll be ready in a few hours. Chia pudding has a creamy consistency, and you can add in fruits, granola, or other typical yogurt toppings.

Closing Thoughts

I hope that, if nothing else, these recipes get your creative mind churning. Making healthy, healing, and delicious food is often much simpler than we expect. Try something new and you may even surprise yourself!

In-Season Produce

God designed the seasons to come and go each year. With that, He also designed the food that thrives in each season to help us thrive in that moment. There's much more that can be written on this topic. For example, different parts of the world experience the seasons differently. There are certainly implications of this. But for this quick reference guide, I'll provide some examples of in-season foods for the typical four seasons. This is by no means an exhaustive list, especially because in-season will look very different by location and climate. In fact, a great resource (which I referenced for the below list) is *seasonalfoodguide.org*. They show in-season produce by location and month. I encourage you to check it out for the area you live in. My hope is that you can continue to see God's design for our food and that eating in-season becomes an exciting challenge instead of a restricting issue (or even a complete unknown).

Why Eat In-Season?

- Buying in-season produce means that you can buy locally much easier. This allows you to know your food source and support the local economy instead of the global food industry.
- In-season produce is easier to grow, likely reducing the need to use synthetic chemicals to be used to keep the crop alive.
- In-season produce can contain higher concentrations of nutrients.
- In-season produce likely isn't shipped internationally and artificially ripened.

Season	Examples of In-Season Fruits	Examples of In-Season Vegetables
Winter	Orange, Grapefruit, Apples, Lemons	Sweet Potatoes, Potatoes, Radish, Butternut Squash, Spaghetti Squash
Spring	Strawberries, Cherries, Pineapple, Avocado	Leafy Greens, Herbs, Onion, Asparagus, Fennel, Radishes, Microgreens (Pea Shoots, Sprouts)
Summer	Blueberries, Strawberries, Raspberries, Cantaloupe, Watermelon	Green Beans, Okra, Summer Squash, Tomatoes, Eggplant
Autumn	Apples, Asian Pears, Raspberries, Dates, Figs	Leafy Greens, Broccoli, Cauliflower, Pumpkin, Bell Peppers

Acknowledgements

Thank You!

There are so many people to thank, not only for helping make this book a reality but also for shaping my life in such a way that *Designed to Heal* was a natural overflow of it.

Thank you to Samantha Gambale, my outstanding editor. Sam perfectly combined her command of the English language with her heart for the Lord in reviewing this book. Without her, *Designed to Heal* would not be the same.

Thank you to Bryan Shadron and Russ Griffith. Both of these men read and provided honest feedback on a very raw version of this book. Their thoughtful comments pointed me in the right direction and helped me to honor God more in my writing.

Thank you to my mom, Cheryl Morgan. As any of my friends from childhood will attest, she cared about real food far before I ever did. She seeks to honor God with her whole life, including how she eats and feeds her family. She is one of my biggest inspirations.

And most of all, thank you to my beautiful, strong, and inspiring wife, Haley. It's taken unbelievable dedication and hard work, but watching you heal has been one of the greatest honors of my life. Now we can look back and see how God used the hardest point in your life to change our lives and the lives of many others. I love you.

Referenced Sources

Chapter 1: The Healing Nature

1. "The Top 10 Fears in America 2022." Chapman University. October 14, 2022. blogs.chapman.edu/wilkinson/2022/10/14/the-top-10-fears-in-america-2022

2. "The Immune System." Johns Hopkins Medicine. Accessed September 17, 2023. www.hopkinsmedicine.org/health/conditions-and-diseases/the-immune-system

Chapter 2: Food Is God's Medicine

1. "U.S. Food Retail Industry—Statistics & Facts." Statista Research Department. January 24, 2022. www.statista.com/topics/1660/food-retail

2. Axe, Josh, DNM. *Ancient Remedies*, Page 70. Hachette Book Group. February 2021.

3. Axe, Josh, DNM. *Ancient Remedies*, Page 101. Hachette Book Group. February 2021.

4. Brazier, Yvette. "What Are Vitamins, and How Do They Work?" Medical News Today. October 5, 2023. www.medicalnewstoday.com/articles/195878

5. Hill, Ansley, RD, LD. "Top 14 Health Benefits of Broccoli." Healthline. September 12, 2018. www.healthline.com/nutrition/benefits-of-broccoli

6. Pandey, Kanti and Syed Rizvi. "Plant Polyphenols as Dietary Antioxidants in Human Health and Disease." Oxidative Medicine and Cellular Longevity. December 2009. www.ncbi.nlm.nih.gov/pmc/articles/PMC2835915

Chapter 3: How We Used to Live

1. Roth, Gregory, MD Et Al. "Global Burden of Cardiovascular Diseases and Risk Factors, 1990–2019: Update from the GBD 2019 Study." Journal of the American College of Cardiology. December 2020. www.jacc.org/doi/10.1016/j.jacc.2020.11.010

2. Liu, Qingqing Et Al. "Changes in the Global Burden of Depression from 1990 to 2017: Findings from the Global Burden of Disease Study." Journal of Psychiatric Research. May 30, 2020. www.doi.org/10.1016/j.jpsychires.2019.08.002

3. Mackay, Ian. "Travels and Travails of Autoimmunity: A Historical Journey from Discovery to Rediscovery." Autoimmunity Reviews. October 31, 2009. www.doi.org/10.1016/j.autrev.2009.10.007

4. "Progress in Autoimmune Disease Research." Page 18. National Institutes of Health. March 2005. www.niaid.nih.gov/sites/default/files/adccfinal.pdf

5. "1-in-5 Brochure." American Autoimmune Related Diseases Association. Accessed September 17, 2023. www.autoimmune.org/wp-content/uploads/2019/12/1-in-5-Brochure.pdf

6. "Chronic Diseases in America." Center for Disease Control. Accessed September 17, 2023. www.cdc.gov/chronicdisease/resources/infographic/chronic-diseases.htm

7. "A Post-Pandemic Look at the State of Loneliness among U.S. Adults." The Cigna Group. Accessed September 17, 2023; newsroom.thecignagroup.com/loneliness-epidemic-persists-post-pandemic-look

8. "Short Sleep Duration Among US Adults." Center for Disease Control. Accessed September 17, 2023. www.cdc.gov/sleep/data_statistics.html

9. "Your Guide to Healthy Sleep." National Heart, Lung, and Blood Institute. January 2011. www.nhlbi.nih.gov/sites/default/files/publications/11-5271.pdf

Chapter 4: Balancing Act

1. Pahwa, Roma Et Al. "Chronic Inflammation." StatPearls Publishing. September 28, 2021. www.ncbi.nlm.nih.gov/books/NBK493173/

2. Hanson, Petra, PhD and Thomas Barber, MD. "Is the Microbiome Another Organ? Maybe We Should Treat It as Such." Medical News Today. May 24, 2021; www.medicalnewstoday.com/articles/is-the-microbiome-another-organ-maybe-we-should-treat-it-like-it-is

3. Bull, Matthew, and Nigel Plummer. "Part 1: The Human Gut Microbiome in Health and Disease." Integrative Medicine (Encinitas, California). December 2014. www.ncbi.nlm.nih.gov/pmc/articles/PMC4566439

4. Satokari, Reetta. "High Intake of Sugar and the Balance between Pro- and Anti-Inflammatory Gut Bacteria." Nutrients. May 8, 2020. www.ncbi.nlm.nih.gov/pmc/articles/PMC7284805

5. Davis, Nicole. "Bugs in the System." Harvard Public Health. Accessed September 17, 2023. www.hsph.harvard.edu/magazine/magazine_article/bugs-in-the-system

Chapter 5: More Than Physical

1. Carpenter, Siri, PhD. "That Gut Feeling." American Psychological Association. September 2012. www.apa.org/monitor/2012/09/gut-feeling

2. Myhre, James and Dennis Sifris, MD. "What Is Glycine?" Very Well Health. August 31, 2023. www.verywellhealth.com/glycine-overview-4583816

3. "The Connection Between Diet and Mental Health." The Center for Treatment of Anxiety and Mood Disorders. Accessed September 17, 2023; www.centerforanxietydisorders.com/diet-and-mental-health

Chapter 6: Chasing Convenience

1. Anderson, Jill. "The Benefit of Family Mealtime." Harvard Graduate School of Education. April 1, 2020. www.gse.harvard.edu/news/20/04/harvard-edcast-benefit-family-mealtime

2. Shaw, William, PhD Et Al. "Stress Effects on the Body." American Psychological Association. March 8, 2023. www.apa.org/topics/stress/body

Chapter 7: Corporate Shortcuts

1. Poti, Jennifer Et Al. "Is the Degree of Food Processing and Convenience Linked with the Nutritional Quality of Foods Purchased by US Households?" The American Journal of Clinical Nutrition. June 2015. www.doi.org/10.3945/ajcn.114.100925

2. "About The Company." PepsiCo. Accessed September 17, 2023; www.pepsico.com.au/about/about-the-company

3. "Processed Foods and Health." Harvard School of Public Health; Accessed September 17, 2023; www.hsph.harvard.edu/nutritionsource/processed-foods

4. Louzada, Maria Et Al. "Impact of Ultra-Processed Foods on Micronutrient Content in the Brazilian Diet." Revista de Saúde Pública. July 30, 2015. www.ncbi.nlm.nih.gov/pmc/articles/PMC4560336

5. Wallinga, David. "Today's Food System: How Healthy Is It?" Journal of Hunger and Environmental Nutrition. July 2009. ncbi.nlm.nih.gov/pmc/articles/PMC3489133

6. "GE Food & Your Health." Center for Food Safety. Accessed September 17, 2023. www.centerforfoodsafety.org/issues/311/ge-foods/ge-food-and-your-health

7. "Prescription Drugs." Georgetown Health Policy Institute. Accessed September 17, 2023. hpi.georgetown.edu/rxdrugs

Chapter 8: Tantalizing Taste

1. Ede, Georgia, MD. "The Brain Needs Animal Fat." Psychology Today. March 31, 2019. www.psychologytoday.com/us/blog/diagnosis-diet/201903/the-brain-needs-animal-fat

2. Winterdahl, Michael Et Al. "Sucrose Intake Lowers μ-Opioid and Dopamine D2/3 Receptor Availability in Porcine Brain." Scientific Reports. November 15, 2019. www.doi.org/10.1038/s41598-019-53430-9

3. Patterson, Danial. "Vegetable Oils: A History of Fats Gone Wrong." Zero Acre Blog. April 10, 2023. www.zeroacre.com/blog/the-history-of-vegetable-oils

4. "Hexane." Environmental Protection Agency. Accessed September 17, 2023; www.epa.gov/sites/default/files/2016-09/documents/hexane.pdf

5. Gritz, Jennie. "The Unsavory History of Sugar, the Insatiable American Craving." Smithsonian Magazine. May 2017. smithsonianmag.com/history/unsavory-history-sugar-american-craving-180962766

6. Desilver, Drew. "What's on Your Table? How America's Diet Has Changed Over the Decades." Pew Research. December 13, 2016. www.pewresearch.org/fact-tank/2016/12/13/whats-on-your-table-how-americas-diet-has-changed-over-the-decades

7. Sung, Heyeon Et Al. "High-Sucrose Diet Exposure is Associated with Selective and Reversible Alterations in the Rat Peripheral Taste System." Current Biology. October 10, 2022. www.doi.org/10.1016/j.cub.2022.07.063

Chapter 9: The Taste Pitch

1. Story, Mary and Simone French. "Food Advertising and Marketing Directed at Children and Adolescents in the US." International Journal of Behavioral Nutrition and Physical Activity. February 10, 2004. www.doi.org/10.1186/1479-5868-1-3

2. Signal, L.N. Et Al. "Children's Everyday Exposure to Food Marketing: An Objective Analysis Using Wearable Cameras." International Journal of Behavioral Nutrition and Physical Activity. October 8, 2017. www.ncbi.nlm.nih.gov/pmc/articles/PMC5632829

3. McKay, Brett and Kate McKay. "Podcast #754: A Surprising Theory on Why We Get Fat." The Art of Manliness. November 8, 2021. www.artofmanliness.com/health-fitness/health/podcast-754-a-surprising-theory-on-why-we-get-fat

4. Myers, Iris. "EWG's Dirty Dozen Guide to Food Chemicals: The Top 12 to Avoid." Environmental Working Group. July 11, 2022. www.ewg.org/consumer-guides/ewgs-dirty-dozen-guide-food-chemicals-top-12-avoid

5. Grocholl, Luke, PhD. "Navigating Natural Flavor Regulations." Sigma-Aldrich. Accessed September 17, 2023. www.sigmaaldrich.com/US/en/technical-documents/technical-article/food-and-beverage-testing-and-manufacturing/flavor-and-fragrance-formulation/navigating-natural-flavor-regulations

6. "Dirty Louisiana: Filthy Results at Dirt Cheap Prices." The Marketing Society. Accessed September 17, 2023. www.marketingsociety.com/sites/default/files/thelibrary/KFC%20winner%20Finance%20Director%27s%20Prize_Redacted1.pdf

Chapter 10: Counting the Costs

1. Fahey, Mark and Nicholas Wells. "Americans Think About Money and Work More Than Sex, Survey Finds." NBC News. September 9, 2015. www.nbcnews.com/better/money/americans-think-about-money-work-more-sex-survey-finds-n424261

2. Gaffigan, Jim. "'That's McDonald's!' - Jim Gaffigan (Mr. Universe)." Jim Gaffigan's Official YouTube Channel. April 9, 2020. www.youtube.com/watch?v=KYKGFujJp6Y&t

3. "Food Prices and Spending." United States Department of Agriculture Economic Research Service. Accessed September 23, 2023. www.ers.usda.gov/data-products/ag-and-food-statistics-charting-the-essentials/food-prices-and-spending

Chapter 11: Corporate Cost-Cutting

1. Koerth, Maggie. "Big Farms Are Getting Bigger and Most Small Farms Aren't Really Farms at All." FiveThirtyEight. November 17, 2016. www.fivethirtyeight.com/features/big-farms-are-getting-bigger-and-most-small-farms-arent-really-farms-at-all

2. "Glyphosate: Response to Comments, Usage, and Benefits." Environmental Protection Agency. April 18, 2019. www.epa.gov/sites/default/files/2019-04/documents/glyphosate-response-comments-usage-benefits-final.pdf

3. "Human Health Issues Related to Pesticides." Environmental Protection Agency. Accessed September 23, 2023. www.epa.gov/pesticide-science-and-assessing-pesticide-risks/human-health-issues-related-pesticides

4. Tu, Pengchang Et Al. "Gut Microbiome Toxicity: Connecting the Environment and Gut Microbiome-Associated Diseases." Toxics. March 12, 2020. www.ncbi.nlm.nih.gov/pmc/articles/PMC7151736

5. Alavanja, Michael Et Al. "Health Effects of Chronic Pesticide Exposure: Cancer and Neurotoxicity." Annual Reviews. April 21, 2004. www.doi.org/10.1146/annurev.publhealth.25.101802.123020

6. Erickson, Britt. "Bayer to End Glyphosate Sales to US consumers." Chemicals and Engineering News. July 30, 2021. cen.acs.org/environment/pesticides/Bayer-end-glyphosate-sales-US/99/web/2021/07

7. Fields, Scott. "The Fat of the Land: Do Agricultural Subsidies Foster Poor Health?" Environmental Health Perspectives. October 2004. www.ncbi.nlm.nih.gov/pmc/articles/PMC1247588

8. Dorning, Mike. "U.S. Farm Profit on Track for Seven-Year High After Trump Aid." Bloomberg. December 2, 2020. www.bloomberg.com/news/articles/2020-12-02/u-s-farm-profit-on-track-for-seven-year-high-after-trump-aid

9. "Farms and Farmland." 2017 Census of Agriculture. Accessed September 17, 2023. www.nass.usda.gov/Publications/highlights/2019/2017Census_Farms_Farmland.pdf

10. "Soy and Corn: Healthy Choices or Hidden Ingredients?!" Co-Op. Accessed September 23, 2023. www.grocery.coop/fresh-from-the-source/soy-and-corn-healthy-choices-or-hidden-ingredients

Chapter 12: The Foundations

1. McEvoy, Miles. "Organic 101: What the USDA Organic Label Means." U.S. Department of Agriculture. March 13, 2019. www.usda.gov/media/blog/2012/03/22/organic-101-what-usda-organic-label-means

2. "EWG's Shopper's Guide to Pesticides in Produce." Environmental Working Group. Accessed September 17, 2023. www.ewg.org/foodnews/dirty-dozen.php

3. Kresser, Chris. "Why Local Trumps Organic for Nutrient Content." October 26, 2012. www.chriskresser.com/why-local-trumps-organic-for-nutrient-content

4. "Shelf Stable Unsweetened Original Almondmilk." Blue Diamond Growers, Almond Breeze. Accessed October 8, 2023. www.bluediamond.com/brand/almond-breeze/shelf-stable-almondmilk/shelf-stable-unsweetened-original-almondmilk

5. Daley, CA Et Al. "A Review of Fatty Acid Profiles and Antioxidant Content in Grass-Fed and Grain-Fed Beef." Nutrition Journal. March 10, 2010. www.ncbi.nlm.nih.gov/pmc/articles/PMC2846864

6. "'Free Range' and 'Pasture Raised' Officially Defined by HFAC for Certified Humane Label." Certified Humane. January 16, 2014. www.certifiedhumane.org/free-range-and-pasture-raised-officially-defined-by-hfac-for-certified-humane-label

7. "Omega-3 Fatty Acids." National Institutes of Health. Accessed September 17, 2023. www.ods.od.nih.gov/factsheets/Omega3FattyAcids-Consumer

8. Beal, Ty and Flaminia Ortenzi. "Priority Micronutrient Density in Foods." Frontiers in Nutrition. March 7, 2022. www.frontiersin.org/articles/10.3389/fnut.2022.806566/full

9. McEvoy, Miles. "Organic 101: What the USDA Organic Label Means." U.S. Department of Agriculture. March 13, 2019. www.usda.gov/media/blog/2012/03/22/organic-101-what-usda-organic-label-means

10. Links, Rachel, MS, RD. "Is Butter Bad for You, or Good?" Healthline. March 14, 2019. www.healthline.com/nutrition/is-butter-bad-for-you

11. Chowdhury, Rajiv Et Al. "Association of Dietary, Circulating, and Supplement Fatty Acids with Coronary Risk: A Systematic Review and Meta-Analysis." Annals of Internal Medicine. March 18, 2014. www.pubmed.ncbi.nlm.nih.gov/24723079

12. Gunnars, Kris, BSc. "Are Vegetable and Seed Oils Bad for Your Health?" Healthline. June 9, 2023. www.healthline.com/nutrition/are-vegetable-and-seed-oils-bad

13. Simopoulos, Artemis. "An Increase in the Omega-6/Omega-3 Fatty Acid Ratio Increases the Risk for Obesity." Nutrients. March 2, 2016. www.pubmed.ncbi.nlm.nih.gov/26950145

14. "EWG's Tap Water Database." Environmental Working Group. Accessed September 18, 2023. www.ewg.org/tapwater

Chapter 13: The Threats

1. "Skittles Original Fruity Candy." Skittles. Accessed August 27, 2023. www.skittles.com/products/skittles-original-fruity-candy-single-pack-217-oz-skittles-chewy

2. "CFR - Code of Federal Regulations Title 21." U.S. Food and Drug Administration. Accessed September 18, 2023. accessdata.fda.gov/scripts/cdrh/cfdocs/cfcfr/cfrsearch.cfm?fr=101.22

3. "Wheat Thins Original Whole Grain Wheat Crackers." Snackworks. Accessed August 27, 2023. www.snackworks.com/product/00044000009625

4. "Simple Mills - Fine Ground Sea Salt Almond Flour Crackers." Simple Mills. Accessed August 27, 2023. www.simplemills.com/Shop/Product/Fine-Ground-Sea-Salt-Almond-Flour-Crackers.aspx

5. "Butylated Hydroxyanisole." U.S. Department of Health and Human Services, Report on Carcinogens, Fifteenth Edition. Accessed September 18, 2023. ntp.niehs.nih.gov/ntp/roc/content/profiles/butylatedhydroxyanisole.pdf

6. "Powerade Mountain Berry Blast." Powerade. Accessed October 8, 2023. www.powerade.com/products/powerade/mountain-berry-blast

7. "Coca-Cola." Coca-Cola. Accessed October 8, 2023. us.coca-cola.com/products/coca-cola/original

8. "Whole Grains." Harvard School of Public Health. Accessed September 18, 2023. www.hsph.harvard.edu/nutritionsource/what-should-you-eat/whole-grains

9. "Sprouted Whole Grain." Oldways Whole Grain Council. Accessed September 18, 2023. www.wholegrainscouncil.org/whole-grains-101/whats-whole-grain-refined-grain/sprouted-whole-grains

10. "Glyphosate Facts Everybody Should Know." Only Organic. February 13, 2020. www.onlyorganic.org/glyphosate-facts-everyone-should-know

11. Liu, Bin Et Al. "Bovine Milk with Variant β-Casein Types on Immunological Mediated Intestinal Changes and Gut Health of Mice." Frontiers In Nutrition. September 30, 2022. www.frontiersin.org/articles/10.3389/fnut.2022.970685/full

Chapter 14: The Lifestyle

1. "53 Real Ingredients." Chipotle. Accessed August 27, 2023. www.chipotle.com/ingredients

2. Seyfried, Thomas, PhD and Dr. Mark Hyman. "A Radical New Dietary Approach to Cancer Treatment." The Doctor's Farmacy Podcast, Episode 739. June 21, 2023. www.drhyman.com/blog/2023/06/21/podcast-ep737

3. "Your Guide to Healthy Sleep." National Heart, Lung, and Blood Institute. January 2011. www.nhlbi.nih.gov/sites/default/files/publications/11-5271.pdf

4. Sears, Margaret Et Al. "Arsenic, Cadmium, Lead, and Mercury in Sweat: A Systematic Review." Journal of Environmental and Public Health. February 22, 2012. www.ncbi.nlm.nih.gov/pmc/articles/PMC3312275

5. "The Dirty Dozen: PEG Compounds and their Contaminants." David Suzuki Foundation. Accessed August 28, 2023. www.davidsuzuki.org/living-green/dirty-dozen-peg-compounds-contaminants

6. Yaghoobi, Reza Et Al. "Evidence for Clinical Use of Honey in Wound Healing as an Anti-Bacterial, Anti-Inflammatory, Anti-Oxidant and Anti-Viral Agent: A Review." Jundishapur Journal of Natural Pharmaceutical Products. August 8, 2013. www.ncbi.nlm.nih.gov/pmc/articles/PMC3941901

About
Alex Morgan

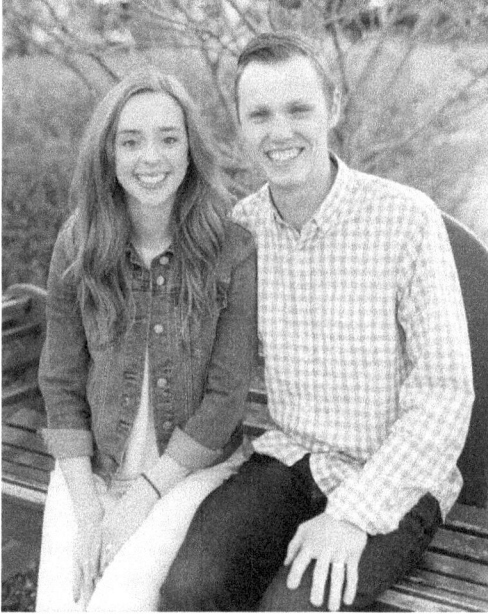

Alex is a disciple of Jesus and husband to Haley. He lives in Charlottesville, Virginia and owns an organic juice and smoothie bar. His passions in life are sharing the good news of the Gospel and helping others flourish in it. This book was written at the intersection of those passions. After witnessing the miracle of Haley's healing through her dedication to eating and enjoying food just how God designed it, he knew he needed to share that experience with others. To connect with Alex, find him on Instagram under the account @designed.2.heal or shoot him an email at designedtoheal23@gmail.com.

www.ingramcontent.com/pod-product-compliance
Lightning Source LLC
Chambersburg PA
CBHW032349280326
41935CB00008B/502